TNM
Classification of Malignant
Tumours

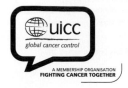

Union for International
Cancer Control (UICC)

TNM
Classification of Malignant Tumours

Eighth Edition

Editors in Chief

James D. Brierley BSc, MB, FRCP, FRCR, FRCPC
Mary K. Gospodarowicz MD, FRCPC, FRCR (Hon)
Christian Wittekind MD

Editors

B. O'Sullivan MD
M. Mason MD
H. Asamura MD
A. Lee MD
E. Van Eycken MD
L. Denny MB, ChB
M.B. Amin MD
S. Gupta MD

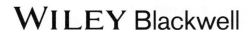

Registered Office
John Wiley & Sons, Ltd, The Atrium, Southern Gate, Chichester, West Sussex, PO19 8SQ, UK

Editorial Offices
9600 Garsington Road, Oxford, OX4 2DQ, UK
111 River Street, Hoboken, NJ 07030, USA

For details of our global editorial offices, customer services, and more information about Wiley products visit us at www.wiley.com.

Wiley also publishes its books in a variety of electronic formats and by print-on-demand. Some content that appears in standard print versions of this book may not be available in other formats.

Library of Congress Cataloging-in-Publication Data

Names: Brierley, James, editor. | Gospodarowicz, M. K. (Mary K.), editor. | Wittekind, Ch. (Christian), editor.
Title: TNM classification of malignant tumours / editors in chief, James D. Brierley, Mary K. Gospodarowicz, Christian Wittekind ; editors, B. O'Sullivan [and 7 others].
Description: Eighth edition. | Oxford, UK ; Hoboken, NJ : John Wiley & Sons, Inc., 2017. | Includes bibliographical references.
Identifiers: LCCN 2016039430 | ISBN 9781119263579 (paper) | ISBN 9781119263548 (Adobe PDF) | ISBN 9781119263562 (epub)
Subjects: | MESH: Neoplasms–classification
Classification: LCC RC258 | NLM QZ 15 | DDC 616.99/40012–dc23
LC record available at https://lccn.loc.gov/2016039430

Cover image: © UICC

Set in 9.25/12pt Joanna MT by SPi Global, Pondicherry, India

10 9 8 7 6 5 4 3 2 1

Editors in Chief

James D. Brierley, BSc, MB, FRCP, FRCR, FRCPC

Professor, Department of Radiation Oncology, University of Toronto; Princess Margaret Cancer Centre, Toronto, Ontario, Canada

Dr Brierley trained in Clinical Oncology in the UK and developed his interest in cancer staging and surveillance when moving to Canada and has been involved in cancer surveillance, locally, nationally and internationally. He is Co-Chair of the UICC TNM Prognostic Factors Project. He has co-edited the TNM Supplement 4th edition (Wiley 2012) and the UICC Manual of Clinical Oncology (Wiley 2015).

Mary K. Gospodarowicz, MD, FRCPC, FRCR (Hon)

Professor, Department of Radiation Oncology, University of Toronto; Medical Director, Princess Margaret Cancer Centre, University Health Network; Regional Vice-President of Cancer Care Ontario for Toronto South, Toronto, Ontario, Canada

Dr Gospodarowicz is the Past-President of UICC. She has a long-standing interest in cancer classification with an emphasis on staging and prognostic factors and she has been involved in the UICC TNM Project for many years. Her interests include the application of modern information and communication technologies in cancer control. Dr Gospodarowicz was co-editor of the 7th edition of the TNM Classification of Malignant Tumours (Wiley 2009) and editor of the 2nd and 3rd editions of the UICC Prognostic Factors in Cancer (Wiley 2001, 2006).

Christian Wittekind, MD

Professor of Pathology, Chairman Institute of Pathology, University of Leipzig, Leipzig, Germany

Dr Wittekind been involved in cancer staging and tumour classifications for over 20 years. He is a member of the UICC TNM Core Committee, Head of the German Speaking TNM-Komittee, and personally responds to all the questions to the UICC TNM helpdesk. He was the co-editor of the 5th, 6th and 7th editions of the TNM Classification of Malignant Tumours (Wiley 1997, 2002, 2009), editor of the 2nd 3rd, and 4th editions of the TNM Supplement (Wiley 2001, 2003 and 2012) and editor of the 6th edition of the TNM Atlas (Wiley 2014).

Editors

B. O'Sullivan, MD
Professor, Department of Radiation Oncology, University of Toronto, Princess Margaret Cancer Centre, Toronto, Ontario, Canada

M. Mason, MD
Professor of Cancer Studies, School of Medicine, Cardiff University, Cardiff, UK

H. Asamura, MD
Professor of Surgery, Chief, Division of Thoracic Surgery, Keio University School of Medicine, Tokyo, Japan

A. Lee, MD
Professor and Head, Department of Clinical Oncology, The University of Hong Kong and the University of Hong Kong-Shenzhen Hospital, Hong Kong, China

E. Van Eycken, MD
Belgian Cancer Registry, Brussels, Belgium

L. Denny, MB, ChB
Head, Department of Obstetrics and Gynaecology, SA Medical Research Council, Gynaecological Cancer Research Centre, Faculty of Health Sciences, University of Cape Town and Groote Schuur Hospital, Cape Town, South Africa

M.B. Amin, MD
Professor and Chair of the Department of Pathology, the College of Medicine, University of Tennessee, Tennessee, USA

S. Gupta, MD
Assistant Professor, Department of Paediatrics, University of Toronto, Division of Haematology/Oncology, Hospital for Sick Children, Toronto, Ontario, Canada

They are called wise
who put things in their right order
Thomas Aquinas

This Eighth Edition is dedicated to Dr Leslie H. Sobin MD, a pathologist and previous long term Chair of UICC TNM Prognostic Factor Committee. Les, as he is known to colleagues all over the world, has devoted most of his career to help promote globally unified classifications of disease in particular in pathology and cancer staging. This is the first edition since the fourth that has not benefitted from his direct involvement; however his imprint is found throughout this edition.

Contents

Preface

In this eighth edition of TNM Classification of Malignant Tumours, many of the tumour sites are unchanged from the seventh edition[1]. However, some tumour entities and anatomic sites have been newly introduced and some tumours contain modifications: this follows the basic philosophy of maintaining stability of the classification over time. The modifications and additions reflect new data on prognosis as well as new methods for assessing prognosis.[2] Some changes had already appeared in the TNM Supplement[3] as proposals. Subsequent support warrants their incorporation into the classification. New proposals for tumours of parathyroid carcinoma, and paraganglionoma will be published in the next edition of the TNM Supplement.

In the seventh edition a new approach was adopted to separate stage groupings from prognostic groupings in which other prognostic factors are added to T, N, and M categories. These new prognostic groupings were presented for oesophagus and prostate. In this eighth edition, the term 'stage' is used when only descriptions of anatomic extent of disease are used and 'prognostic group' for when additional prognostic factors are incorporated.

Changes made between the seventh and eighth editions are indicated by a bar at the left-hand side of the text. To avoid ambiguity, users are encouraged to cite the edition and year of the TNM publication they have used in their list of references.

A TNM homepage with Frequently Asked Questions (FAQs) and a form for submitting questions or comments on the TNM can be found at: http://www.uicc.org.

The UICC's TNM Prognostic Factors Project has a process for evaluating proposals to change the TNM Classification. This procedure aims at a continuous systematic approach composed of two arms: (1) review formal proposals from investigators and (2) an annual literature search for articles concerning improvements to TNM. The proposals and results of the literature search are evaluated by a UICC panel of experts as well as by the TNM Prognostic Factors committee members.[5] The national TNM Committees participated in this process. More details and a checklist that will facilitate the formulation of proposals can be obtained at www.uicc.org.

Union for International Cancer Control (UICC)
62, route de Frontenex
CH-1207 Geneva, Switzerland
Fax +41 22 8091810

References

1 Sobin LH, Gospodarowicz MK, Wittekind Ch., eds. *International Union Against Cancer (UICC). TNM Classification of Malignant Tumours*, 7th edn. New York: Wiley, 2009.
2 Gospodarowicz MK, O'Sullivan B, Sobin LH, eds. *International Union Against Cancer (UICC): Prognostic Factors in Cancer*, 3rd edn. New York: Wiley, 2006.
3 Wittekind Ch, Compton CC, Brierley J, Sobin LH, eds. *International Union Against Cancer (UICC): TNM Supplement. A Commentary on Uniform Use*, 4th edn. Oxford: Wiley Blackwell Publications, 2012.
4 Amin MB, Edge SB, Greene FL, et al., eds. *American Joint Committee on Cancer (AJCC) Cancer Staging Manual*, 8th edn. New York: Springer, 2017.
5 Webber C, Gospodawowicz M, Sobin LH, et al. Improving the TNM Classification: findings from a 10 year continuous literature review. *Int J Cancer* 2014; 135: 371–378.

Acknowledgments

The Editors have much pleasure in acknowledging the great help received from the members of the TNM Prognostic Factors Project Committee and the National Staging Committees Global Representatives and international organizations listed on pages XVI, all of whom volunteered their time.

We thank Professor Patti Groome and Ms Colleen Webber for supervising and performing the literature watch from its inception until 2015 and 2016, respectively. The eighth edition of the TNM *Classification* is the result of a number of consultative meetings organized and supported by the UICC and AJCC secretariats.

This publication was made possible by grants 1U58DP001818 and 1U58DP004965 from the Centers for Disease Control and Prevention (CDC) (USA). Its contents are solely the responsibility of the authors and do not necessarily represent the official views of the CDC.

Organizations Associated with the TNM System

CDC	Centers for Disease Control and Prevention (USA)
FIGO	International Federation of Gynaecology and Obstetrics
IACR	International Association of Cancer Registries
IARC	International Agency for Research on Cancer
IASLC	International Association for the Study of Lung Cancer
ICCR	International Collaboration on Cancer Reporting
WHO	World Health Organization

National Committees

Australia and New Zealand	National TNM Committee
Austria, Germany, Switzerland	Deutschsprachiges TNM-Komitee
Belgium	National TNM Committee
Brazil	National TNM Committee
Canada	National Staging Steering Committee
China	National TNM Cancer Staging Committee of China
Denmark	National TNM Committee
Gulf States	TNM Committee
India	National TNM Committee
Israel	National Cancer Staging Committee
Italy	Italian Prognostic Systems Project
Japan	Japanese Joint Committee
Latin America and Caribbean	Sociedad Latinoamericana y del Caribe de Oncología Médica
Netherlands	National Staging Committee
Poland	National Staging Committee
Singapore	National Staging Committee
Spain	National Staging Committee
South Africa	National Staging Committee
Turkey	Turkish National Cancer Staging Committee
United Kingdom	National Staging Committee
United States of America	American Joint Committee on Cancer

Members of UICC Committees Associated with the TNM System

In 1950 the UICC appointed a *Committee on Tumour Nomenclature and Statistics*. In 1954 this Committee became known as the *Committee on Clinical Stage Classification and Applied Statistics* and in 1966 it was named the *Committee on TNM Classification*. Taking into consideration new prognostic factors the Committee was named in 1994 the *TNM Prognostic Factors Project Committee*, and in 2003 the main committee was named "TNM Prognostic Factors Core Group". A list of members who have served on these committees is available at: www.uicc.org

UICC TNM Prognostic Factors Core Group 2016

Asamura, H.	Japan
Brierley, J.D.	Canada
Compton, C.C.	USA
Gospodarowicz, M.K.	Canada
Lee, Anne	China
Mason, M.	UK
O'Sullivan, B.	Canada
Van Eycken, E.	Belgium
Wittekind, Ch.	Germany

Section Editors

General Rules	J.D. Brierley
	M. K. Gospodarowicz
	B. O'Sullivan
	Ch. Wittekind
Head and Neck	B. O'Sullivan
Thyroid	J.D. Brierley
Upper Gastrointestinal Tract	Ch. Wittekind
Lower Gastrointestinal Tract	J.D. Brierley
Hepatobiliary	Ch. Wittekind
Lung, Pleura and Thymic Tumours	H. Asamura
Bone and Soft Tissues	B. O'Sullivan
Skin	A. Lee, J.D. Brierley, B. O'Sullivan
Breast	E. Van Eckyen
Gynecological	L. Denny
Genitourinary	M.K. Gospodarowicz, M. Mason
Ophthalmic Tumours	Ch. Wittekind
Malignant Lymphoma	M.K. Gospodarowicz
Paediatric Tumours	S. Gupta, J.D. Brierley
Essential TNM	J.D. Brierley, B. O'Sullivan
AJCC Liaison	M.B. Amin

In addition, the Editors wish to acknowledge the invaluable contributions of:

Head and Neck Cancers	UICC Advisory Committee (see www.uicc.org)
Thymic Tumours	F. Detterbeck
Cutaneous Squamous Cell Carcinoma	C. Schmults, K. Nehal
Essential TNM	F. Bray, M. Parkin, M. Pineros, K. Ward, M. Ervik, A. Znaor
Paediatric Tumours	L. Frazier, J. Aitken
Expert Panel Members	See www.uicc.org
Global Advisory Group Members	See www.uicc.org

Introduction

The History of the TNM System*

The TNM system for the classification of malignant tumours was developed by Pierre Denoix (France) between the years 1943 and 1952.[1]

In 1950, the UICC appointed a Committee on Tumour Nomenclature and Statistics. As a basis for its work on clinical stage classification, it adopted the general definitions of local extension of malignant tumours suggested by the World Health Organization (WHO) Sub-Committee on The Registration of Cases of Cancer as well as Their Statistical Presentation.[2]

In 1958, the Committee published the first recommendations for the clinical stage classification of cancers of the breast and larynx and for the presentation of results.[3]

A second publication in 1959 presented revised proposals for the breast, for clinical use and evaluation over a 5-year period (1960–1964).[4] In 1968, a booklet, the *Livre de Poche*[5] and, a year later, a complementary booklet was published detailing recommendations for the setting-up of field trials, for the presentation of end results, and for the determination and expression of cancer survival rates.[6] The *Livre de Poche* was subsequently translated into 11 languages. In 1974 and 1978, second and third editions[7,8] were published containing new site classifications, and the fourth edition of TNM in 1987.[9]

In 1993, the project published the *TNM Supplement*[10] to promote the uniform use of TNM by providing detailed explanations of the TNM rules with practical examples. Second, third, and fourth editions appeared in 2001, 2003, and 2012.[11–13]

The project also publishes the *TNM Atlas an Illustrated Guide to the TNM Classification of Malignant Tumours*, the sixth edition was published in 2014 as a companion to the seventh edition of the TNM Classification.[14]

In 1995, the project published *Prognostic Factors in Cancer*,[15] a compilation and discussion of prognostic factors in cancer, both anatomical and non-anatomical, at each of the body sites. This was expanded in the second edition in 2001[16] and the third edition in 2006.[17]

The current eighth edition of TNM contains rules of classification and staging that correspond with those appearing in the eighth edition of the *AJCC Cancer Staging Manual* (2017).[18] While the aim of the UICC and AJCC is to have identical classifications, small differences exist and are identified as footnotes to the text. Wherever possible, the UICC classification is based on published evidence-based recommendation.

To develop and sustain a classification system acceptable to all requires the closest liaison between national and international organizations. As noted, while the classification is based on published evidence, in areas where high-level evidence is not available it is based on international consensus. The continuing objective of the UICC is to present the classification of anatomical extent of cancer globally.

Note
* A more detailed history is available on the website at www.uicc.org

The Principles of the TNM System

The practice of classifying cancer cases into groups according to anatomical extent, termed 'stage', arose from the observation that survival rates were higher for cases in which the disease was localized than for those in which the disease had extended beyond the organ of origin. The stage of disease at the time of diagnosis is a reflection not only of the rate of growth and extension of the neoplasm but also the type of tumour and the tumour–host relationship.

It is important to record accurate information on the anatomical extent of the disease for each site at the time of diagnosis, to meet the following objectives:
1. to aid the clinician in the planning of treatment
2. to give some indication of prognosis for survival
3. to assist in evaluation of the results of treatment
4. to facilitate the exchange of information between treatment centres
5. to contribute to the continuing investigation of human cancer
6. to support cancer control activities.

Cancer staging is essential to patient care, research, and cancer control. Cancer control activities include direct patient care-related activities, the development and implementation of clinical practice guidelines, and centralized activities such as recording disease extent in cancer registries for surveillance purposes and planning cancer systems. Recording of stage is essential for the evaluation of outcomes of clinical practice and cancer programmes. However, in order to evaluate the long-term outcomes of populations, it is important for the classification to remain stable. There is therefore a conflict between a classification that is updated to include the most current forms of medical knowledge while also maintaining a classification that facilitating longitudinal studies. The UICC TNM Project aims to address both needs.

International agreement on the classification of cancer by extent of disease provides a method of conveying disease extent to others without ambiguity.

There are many axes of tumour classification: for example, the anatomical site and the clinical and pathological extent of disease, the duration of symptoms or signs, the gender and age of the patient, and the histological type and grade of the tumour. All of these have an influence on the outcome of the disease. Classification by anatomical extent of disease is the one with which the TNM system primarily deals.

The clinician's immediate task when meeting a patient with a new diagnosis of cancer is to make a judgment as to prognosis and a decision as to the most effective course of treatment. This judgment and this decision require, among other things, an objective assessment of the anatomical extent of the disease.

To meet the stated objectives a system of classification is needed:

1. that is applicable to all sites regardless of treatment; and
2. that may be supplemented later by further information that becomes available from histopathology and/or surgery.

The TNM system meets these requirements.

The General Rules of the TNM System[a,b]

The TNM system for describing the anatomical extent of disease is based on the assessment of three components:

T – the extent of the primary tumour
N– the absence or presence and extent of regional lymph node metastasis
M – the absence or presence of distant metastasis.

The addition of numbers to these three components indicates the extent of the malignant disease, thus:

T0, T1, T2, T3, T4, N0, N1, N2, N3, M0, M1

In effect, the system is a 'shorthand notation' for describing the extent of a particular malignant tumour.

The general rules applicable to all sites are as follows:

1. All cases should be confirmed microscopically. Any cases not so proved must be reported separately.
2. Two classifications are described for each site, namely:
   a) *Clinical classification:* the pretreatment clinical classification) designated **TNM** (or cTNM) is essential to select and evaluate therapy. This is based on evidence acquired before treatment. Such evidence is gathered from physical examination, imaging, endoscopy, biopsy, surgical exploration, and other relevant examinations.
   b) *Pathological classification:* the postsurgical histopathological classification, designated **pTNM**, is used to guide adjuvant therapy and provides additional data to estimate prognosis and end results. This is based on evidence acquired before treatment, supplemented or modified by additional evidence acquired from surgery and from pathological examination. The pathological assessment of the primary tumour (pT) entails a resection of the primary tumour or biopsy adequate to evaluate the highest pT category. The pathological assessment of the regional lymph nodes (pN) entails removal of the lymph nodes adequate to validate the absence of regional lymph node metastasis (pN0) or sufficient to evaluate the highest pN category. An excisional biopsy of a lymph node without pathological assessment of the primary is insufficient to fully evaluate the pN category and is a clinical classification. The pathological assessment of distant metastasis (pM) entails microscopic examination of metastatic deposit.
3. After assigning T, N, and M and/or pT, pN, and pM categories, these may be grouped into stages. The TNM classification and stages, are established at diagnosis and must remain unchanged in the medical records.

   Only for cancer surveillance purposes, clinical and pathological data may be combined when only partial information is available either in the pathological classification or the clinical classification.
4. If there is doubt concerning the correct T, N, or M category to which a particular case should be allotted, then the lower (i.e., less advanced) category should be chosen. This will also be reflected in the stage.

5. In the case of multiple primary tumours in one organ, the tumour with the highest T category should be classified and the multiplicity or the number of tumours should be indicated in parenthesis, e.g., T2(m) or T2(5). In simultaneous bilateral primary cancers of paired organs, each tumour should be classified independently. In tumours of the liver, ovary and fallopian tube, multiplicity is a criterion of T classification, and in tumours of the lung multiplicity may be a criterion of the M classification.

6. Definitions of the TNM categories and stage may be telescoped or expanded for clinical or research purposes as long as the basic definitions recommended are not changed. For instance, any T, N, or M can be divided into subgroups.

Notes

[a] For more details on classification the reader is referred to the TNM Supplement.

[b] An educational module is available on the UICC website www.uicc.org.

Anatomical Regions and Sites

The sites in this classification are listed by code number of the International Classification of Diseases for Oncology.[19] Each region or site is described under the following headings:

- Rules for classification with the procedures for assessing the T, N, and M categories
- Anatomical sites, and subsites if appropriate
- Definition of the regional lymph nodes
- TNM Clinical classification
- pTNM Pathological classification
- G Histopathological grading if different from that described on page 9
- Stage and prognostic groups
- Prognostic factors grid

TNM Clinical Classification

The following general definitions are used throughout:

T – Primary Tumour

TX	Primary tumour cannot be assessed
T0	No evidence of primary tumour
Tis	Carcinoma in situ
T1–T4	Increasing size and/or local extent of the primary tumour

N – Regional Lymph Nodes

NX   Regional lymph nodes cannot be assessed
N0   No regional lymph node metastasis
N1–N3 Increasing involvement of regional lymph nodes

M – Distant Metastasis*

M0 No distant metastasis
M1 Distant metastasis

Note
* The MX category is considered to be inappropriate as clinical assessment of metastasis can be based on physical examination alone. (The use of MX may result in exclusion from staging.)

The category M1 may be further specified according to the following notation:

Pulmonary	PUL (C34)	Bone marrow	MAR (C42.1)
Osseous	OSS (C40, 41)	Pleura	PLE (C38.4)
Hepatic	HEP (C22)	Peritoneum	PER (C48.1,2)
Brain	BRA (C71)	Adrenals	ADR (C74)
Lymph nodes	LYM (C77)	Skin	SKI (C44)
Others	OTH		

Subdivisions of TNM

Subdivisions of some main categories are available for those who need greater specificity (e.g., T1a, T1b or N2a, N2b).

pTNM Pathological Classification

The following general definitions are used throughout:

pT – Primary Tumour

pTX   Primary tumour cannot be assessed histologically
pT0   No histological evidence of primary tumour
pTis   Carcinoma in situ
pT1–4 Increasing size and/or local extent of the primary tumour histologically

pN – Regional Lymph Nodes

pNX   Regional lymph nodes cannot be assessed histologically
pN0   No regional lymph node metastasis histologically
pN1–3   Increasing involvement of regional lymph nodes histologically

Notes

- Direct extension of the primary tumour into lymph nodes is classified as lymph node metastasis.
- Tumour deposits (satellites), i.e., macro- or microscopic nests or nodules, in the lymph drainage area of a primary carcinoma without histological evidence of residual lymph node in the nodule, may represent discontinuous spread, venous invasion (V1/2) or a totally replaced lymph node. If a nodule is considered by the pathologist to be a totally replaced lymph node (generally having a smooth contour), it should be recorded as a positive lymph node, and each such nodule should be counted separately as a lymph node in the final pN determination.
- Metastasis in any lymph node other than regional is classified as a distant metastasis.
- When size is a criterion for pN classification, measurement is made of the metastasis, not of the entire lymph node. The measurement should be that of the largest dimension of the tumour.
- Cases with micrometastasis only, i.e., no metastasis larger than 0.2 cm, can be identified by the addition of '(mi)', e.g., pN1(mi).

Sentinel Lymph Node

The sentinel lymph node is the first lymph node to receive lymphatic drainage from a primary tumour. If it contains metastatic tumour this indicates that other lymph nodes may contain tumour. If it does not contain metastatic tumour, other lymph nodes are not likely to contain tumour. Occasionally, there is more than one sentinel lymph node.

The following designations are applicable when sentinel lymph node assessment is attempted:

(p)NX(sn)   Sentinel lymph node could not be assessed
(p)N0(sn)   No sentinel lymph node metastasis
(p)N1(sn)   Sentinel lymph node metastasis

Isolated Tumour Cells

Isolated tumour cells (ITC) are single tumour cells or small clusters of cells not more than 0.2 mm in greatest extent that can be detected by routine H and E stains or immunohistochemistry. An additional criterion has been proposed in breast cancer to include a cluster of fewer than 200 cells in a single histological cross-section. Others have proposed for other tumour sites that a cluster should have 20 cells or fewer; definitions of ITC may vary by tumour site. ITCs do not typically show evidence of metastatic activity (e.g., proliferation or stromal reaction) or penetration of vascular or lymphatic sinus walls. Cases with ITC in lymph nodes or at distant sites should be classified as N0 or M0, respectively. The same applies to cases with findings suggestive of tumour cells or their components by non-morphological techniques such as flow cytometry or DNA analysis. The exceptions are in malignant melanoma of the skin and Merkel cell carcinoma, wherein ITC in a lymph node are classified as N1. These cases should be analysed separately.[20] Their classification is as follows.

(p)N0	No regional lymph node metastasis histologically, no examination for isolated tumour cells (ITC)
(p)N0(i–)	No regional lymph node metastasis histologically, negative morphological findings for ITC
(p)N0(i+)	No regional lymph node metastasis histologically, positive morphological findings for ITC
(p)N0(mol–)	No regional lymph node metastasis histologically, negative non-morphological findings for ITC
(p)N0(mol+)	No regional lymph node metastasis histologically, positive non-morphological findings for ITC

Cases with or examined for isolated tumour cells (ITC) in sentinel lymph nodes can be classified as follows:

(p)N0(i–)(sn)	No sentinel lymph node metastasis histologically, negative morphological findings for ITC
(p)N0(i+)(sn)	No sentinel lymph node metastasis histologically, positive morphological findings for ITC
(p)N0(mol–)(sn)	No sentinel lymph node metastasis histologically, negative non-morphological findings for ITC
(p)N0 (mol+)(sn)	No sentinel lymph node metastasis histologically, positive non-morphological findings for ITC

pM – Distant Metastasis*

pM1   Distant metastasis microscopically confirmed

Note

* pM0 and pMX are not valid categories.

The category pM1 may be further specified in the same way as M1 (see page 6).

Isolated tumour cells found in bone marrow with morphological techniques are classified according to the scheme for N, e.g., M0(i+). For non-morphological findings 'mol' is used in addition to M0, e.g., M0 (mol+).

Histopathological Grading

In most sites, further information regarding the primary tumour may be recorded under the following heading:

G – Histopathological Grading

GX   Grade of differentiation cannot be assessed
G1   Well differentiated
G2   Moderately differentiated
G3   Poorly differentiated
G4   Undifferentiated

Notes
- Grades 3 and 4 can be combined in some circumstances as 'G3-4, poorly differentiated or undifferentiated'.
- Special systems of grading are recommended for tumours of breast, corpus uteri, and prostate.

Additional Descriptors

For identification of special cases in the TNM or pTNM classification, the m, y, r, and a symbols may be used. Although they do not affect the stage grouping, they indicate cases needing separate analysis.

m Symbol. The suffix m, in parentheses, is used to indicate the presence of multiple primary tumours at a single site. See TNM rule no. 5.

y Symbol. In those cases in which classification is performed during or following multimodality therapy, the cTNM or pTNM category is identified by a y prefix. The ycTNM or ypTNM categorizes the extent of tumour actually present at the time of that examination. The y categorization is not an estimate of the extent of tumour prior to multimodality therapy.

r Symbol. Recurrent tumours, when classified after a disease-free interval, are identified by the prefix r.

a Symbol. The prefix a indicates that classification is first determined at autopsy.

Optional Descriptors

L – Lymphatic Invasion

LX   Lymphatic invasion cannot be assessed
L0   No lymphatic invasion
L1   Lymphatic invasion

V – Venous Invasion

VX   Venous invasion cannot be assessed
V0   No venous invasion
V1   Microscopic venous invasion
V2   Macroscopic venous invasion

Note
Macroscopic involvement of the wall of veins (with no tumour within the veins) is classified as V2.

Pn – Perineural Invasion

PnX   Perineural invasion cannot be assessed
Pn0   No perineural invasion
Pn1   Perineural invasion

Residual Tumour (R) Classification*

The absence or presence of residual tumour after treatment is described by the symbol R. More details can be found in the TNM Supplement (see Preface, Reference 3).

TNM and pTNM describe the anatomical extent of cancer in general without considering treatment. They can be supplemented by the R classification, which deals with tumour status after treatment. It reflects the effects of therapy, influences further therapeutic procedures, and is a strong predictor of prognosis.

The definitions of the R categories are:

RX   Presence of residual tumour cannot be assessed
R0   No residual tumour
R1   Microscopic residual tumour
R2   Macroscopic residual tumour.

Note
* Some consider the R classification to apply only to the primary tumour and its local or regional extent. Others have applied it more broadly to include distant metastasis. The specific usage should be indicated when the R is used.

Stage and Prognostic Groups

The TNM system is used to describe and record the anatomical extent of disease. For purposes of tabulation and analysis it is useful to condense these categories into groups. For consistency, in the TNM system, carcinoma in situ is categorized stage 0; in general, tumours localized to the organ of origin as stages I and II, locally extensive spread, particularly to regional lymph nodes as stage III, and those with distant metastasis as stage IV. The stage adopted is such as to ensure, as far as possible, that each group is more or less homogeneous in respect of survival, and that the survival rates of these groups for each cancer site are distinctive.

For pathological stages, if sufficient tissue has been removed for pathological examination to evaluate the highest T and N categories, M1 may be either clinical (cM1) or pathological (pM1). However, if only a distant metastasis has had microscopic confirmation, the classification is pathological (pM1) and the stage is pathological.

Although the anatomical extent of disease, as categorized by TNM, is a very powerful prognostic indicator in cancer, it is recognized that many factors have a significant impact on predicting outcomes. This has resulted in different stage groups. In thyroid cancer there are different stage definitions for different histologies and, new to this edition, in oropharyngeal cancer HPV-related cancer is staged differently from non-HPV-related cancer. Some factors have been combined with TNM in the development of stage groupings; for instance, for different histologies (thyroid), different major prognostic factor groups (age in thyroid), and by aetiology (HPV-related oropharyngeal cancer). In this edition the term **stage** has been used as defining the anatomical extent of disease while **prognostic group** for classifications that incorporate other prognostic factors. Historically, age in differentiated thyroid cancer and grade in soft tissue sarcoma are combined with anatomical extent of disease to determine stage, and stage is retained rather than prognostic group in these two sites.

Prognostic Factors Classification

Prognostic factors can be classified as those pertaining to:

- **Anatomic extent of disease:** describes the extent of disease in the patient at the time of diagnosis. Classically, this is TNM but may also include tumour markers that reflect tumour burden, for instance prostate-specific antigen (PSA) in prostate carcinoma or carcinoembryonic antigen (CEA) in colorectal carcinoma.
- **Tumour profile:** this includes pathological (i.e., grade) and molecular features of a tumour, and gene expression patterns that reflect behaviour. These can be:
  - predictive factors
  - prognostic factors
  - companion diagnostic marker.
- **Patient profile:** this includes terms related to the host of the cancer. These can be demographic factors, such as age and gender, or acquired, such as immunodeficiency and performance status.
- **Environment:** this may include treatment-related and education (expertise, access, ageism, and healthcare delivery) and quality of management.

When describing prognostic factors it is important to state what outcome the factors are prognostic for, and at what point in the patient trajectory. Anatomical extent of disease as described by TNM stage defines prognosis for survival.

In the second edition of the UICC *TNM Classification of Malignant Tumours* for each tumour site, grids were developed that identified prognostic factors for survival at time of diagnosis and whether they were considered to be essential, additional, or new and promising.[16] The grids were updated for the third edition[17] and have been further updated and incorporated into the ninth edition of the UICC *Manual of Clinical Oncology*.[21] Essential factors are those that are required in addition to anatomical extent of disease to determine treatment as identified by published clinical practice guidelines. The table is a generic example of the prognostic factors summary grid. The grids from the ninth edition of the UICC *Manual of Clinical Oncology* are reproduced in this eighth edition. Grids are not available for some of the less common tumours.

Examples of the UICC prognostic factors summary 'grid'

Prognostic factors	Tumour related	Host related	Environment related
Essential*	Anatomical disease extent	Age	Availability of access to radiotherapy
Additional	Histological type Tumour bulk Tumour marker level Programmed death 1 (PD-1) receptor and its ligands (PD-L1)	Race Gender Cardiac function	Expertise of a treatment at the specific level (e.g., surgery or radiotherapy)
New and promising	Epidermal growth factor receptor Gene expression patterns	Germline p53	Access to information

* The origin of essential factors as imperatives for treatment decisions are from known and available clinical practice guidelines.

Source: UICC Manual of Clinical Oncology, Ninth Edition. Edited by Brian O'Sullivan, James D. Brierley, Anil K. D'Cruz, Martin F. Fey, Raphael Pollock, Jan B. Vermorken and Shao Hui Huang. © 2015 UICC. Published 2015 by John Wiley & Sons, Ltd.

Essential TNM

Information on anatomical extent of disease at presentation or stage is central to cancer surveillance to determine cancer burden as it provides additional valuable information to incidence and mortality data.[22] However, cancer registries in low and middle income countries frequently have insufficient information to determine complete TNM data, either because of inability to perform necessary investigations or because of lack of recording of information. In view of this, the UICC TNM Project has with the International Agency for Research in Cancer and the National Cancer Institute developed a new classification system 'Essential TNM' that can be used to collect stage data when complete information is not available. To date, Essential TNM schemas have been developed for breast, cervix, colon, and prostate cancer, and are presented in this edition and available for download at www.uicc.org.

Paediatric Tumours

Since the fourth edition, the UICC TNM Classification of Malignant Tumours has not incorporated any classifications of paediatric tumours. This decision has stemmed from the lack of an international standard staging system for many paediatric tumours. To enable stage data collection by population-based cancer registries there needs to be agreement on cancer staging. Recognition of this led to a consensus meeting held in 2014 and resulted in the publication of recommendations on the staging of paediatric malignancies for the purposes of population surveillance.[23] The classifications published are not intended to replace the classifications used by the clinician when treating an individual patient but instead to facilitate the collection of stage by population-based cancer registries.

Related Classifications

Since 1958, WHO has been involved in a programme aimed at providing internationally acceptable criteria for the histological diagnosis of tumours. This has resulted in the *International Histological Classification of Tumours*, which contains, in an illustrated multivolume series, definitions of tumour types and a proposed nomenclature. A new series, *WHO Classification of Tumours − Pathology and Genetics of Tumours*, continues this effort. (Information on these publications is at www.iarc.fr).

The *WHO International Classification of Diseases for Oncology* (ICD-O-3)[19] is a coding system for neoplasms by topography and morphology and for indicating behaviour (e.g., malignant, benign). This coded nomenclature is identical in the morphology field for neoplasms to the Systematized Nomenclature of Medicine (SNOMED).[24]

In the interest of promoting national and international collaboration in cancer research and specifically of facilitating cooperation in clinical investigations, it is recommended that the WHO *Classification of Tumours* be used for classification and definition of tumour types and that the ICD-O-3 code be used for storage and retrieval of data.

References

1 Denoix PF. Nomenclature des cancer. *Bull Inst Nat Hyg* (Paris) 1944: 69−73; 1945: 82−84; 1950: 81−84; 1952: 743−748.

2 World Health Organization. *Technical Report Series*, number 53, July 1952, pp. 47−48.

3 International Union Against Cancer (UICC) Committee on Clinical Stage Classification and Applied Statistics. *Clinical Stage Classification and Presentation of Results, Malignant Tumours of the Breast and Larynx*. Paris, 1958.

4 International Union Against Cancer (UICC) Committee on Stage Classification and Applied Statistics. *Clinical Stage Classification and Presentation of Results, Malignant Tumours of the Breast*. Paris, 1959.

5 International Union Against Cancer (UICC). *TNM Classification of Malignant Tumours*. Geneva, 1968.

6 International Union Against Cancer (UICC). TNM *General Rules*. Geneva, 1969.

7 International Union Against Cancer (UICC). TNM *Classification of Malignant Tumours*, 2nd edn. Geneva, 1974.

8 International Union Against Cancer (UICC) Harmer MH, ed. TNM *Classification of Malignant Tumours*, 3rd edn. Geneva, 1978. (Enlarged and revised 1982.)

9 International Union Against Cancer (UICC) Hermanek P, Sobin LH, eds. TNM *Classification of Malignant Tumours*, 4th edn. Berlin, Heidelberg, New York: Springer Verlag, 1987. (Revised 1992.)

10 International Union Against Cancer (UICC) Hermanek P, Henson DE, Hutter RVP, Sobin LH, eds. TNM *Supplement. A Commentary on Uniform Use*. Berlin, Heidelberg, New York: Springer Verlag, 1993.

11 International Union Against Cancer (UICC) Wittekind Ch, Henson DE, Hutter RVP, Sobin LH, eds. TNM *Supplement. A Commentary on Uniform Use*, 2nd edn. New York: Wiley, 2001.

12 International Union Against Cancer (UICC) Wittekind Ch, Green FL, Henson DE, Hutter RVP, Sobin LH, eds. TNM *Supplement. A Commentary on Uniform Use*, 3rd edn. New York: Wiley, 2003.

13 International Union Against Cancer (UICC) Wittekind Ch, Compton CC., Brierley JD, D.Sobin LH, eds. TNM *Supplement. A Commentary on Uniform Use*, 4th edn. New York: Wiley, 2012.

14 Wittekind Ch, Asamura H, Sobin LH, eds.TNM *Atlas: Illustrated Guide to the TNM Classification of Malignant Tumours*, 6th edn. New York; Wiley, 2014.

15 International Union Against Cancer (UICC) Hermanek P, Gospodarowicz MK, Henson DE, Hutter RVP, Sobin LH, eds. *Prognostic Factors in Cancer*. Berlin, Heidelberg, New York: Springer Verlag, 1995.

16 International Union Against Cancer (UICC) Gospodarowicz MK, Henson DE, Hutter RVP, et al., eds. *Prognostic Factors in Cancer*, 2nd edn. New York: Wiley, 2001.

17 International Union Against Cancer (UICC) Gospodarowicz MK, O'Sullivan B, Sobin LH, eds. *Prognostic Factors in Cancer*, 3rd edn. New York: Wiley, 2006.

18 American Joint Committee on Cancer (AJCC) Amin MB, Edge SB, Greene FL, et al., eds. *Cancer Staging Manual*, 8th edn. New York: Springer, 2017.

19 Fritz A, Percy C, Jack A, Shanmugaratnam K, Sobin L, Parkin DM, Whelan S, eds. *WHO International Classification of Diseases for Oncology ICD-O*, 3rd edn. Geneva: WHO, 2000.

20 Hermanek P, Hutter RVP, Sobin LH, Wittekind Ch. Classification of isolated tumour cells and micrometastasis. *Cancer* 1999; 86: 2668–2673.

21 O'Sullivan B, Brierley J, D'Cruz A, Fey M, Pollock R, Vermorken J, Huang S. *Manual of Clinical Oncology*, 9th edn. Oxford: Wiley-Blackwell, 2015.

22 The World Health Organization. *Cancer Control Knowledge into Action, Guide for Effective Programs*. Available at: www.who.int/cancer/modules/en/ (accessed Aug. 2016).

23 Gupta S, Aitken J, Bartels U, et al. Paediatric cancer stage in population-based cancer registries: the Toronto consensus principles and guidelines. *Lancet Oncol* 2016; 17: e163–172.

24 SNOMED International: *The Systematized Nomenclature of Human and Veterinary Medicine*. Northfield, Ill: College of American Pathologists. Available at: www.cap.org (accessed Aug. 2016).

Head and Neck Tumours

Introductory Notes

The following sites are included:
- Lip and oral cavity
- Pharynx: oropharynx (p16 negative and p16 positive), nasopharynx, hypopharynx
- Larynx: supraglottis, glottis, subglottis
- Nasal cavity and paranasal sinuses (maxillary and ethmoid sinus)
- Unknown primary carcinoma – cervical nodes
- Malignant melanoma of upper aerodigestive tract
- Major salivary glands
- Thyroid gland

Carcinomas arising in minor salivary glands of the upper aerodigestive tract are classified according to the rules for tumours of their anatomic site of origin, e.g., oral cavity.

Each site is described under the following headings:
- Rules for classification with the procedures for assessing T, N, and M categories; additional methods may be used when they enhance the accuracy of appraisal before treatment
- Anatomical sites and subsites where appropriate
- Definition of the regional lymph nodes
- TNM clinical classification
- pTNM pathological classification
- Stage
- Prognostic factors grid.

Regional Lymph Nodes

Midline nodes are considered ipsilateral nodes except in the thyroid.

TNM *Classification of Malignant Tumours*, Eighth Edition. Edited by James D. Brierley,
Mary K. Gospodarowicz and Christian Wittekind.
© 2017 UICC. Published 2017 by John Wiley & Sons, Ltd.

Lip and Oral Cavity
(ICD-O-3 C00, C02-006)

Rules for Classification

The classification applies only to carcinomas of the vermilion surfaces of the lips and of the oral cavity, including those of minor salivary glands. There should be histological confirmation of the disease.

The following are the procedures for assessing T, N, and M categories:

T *categories*	Physical examination and imaging
N *categories*	Physical examination and imaging
M *categories*	Physical examination and imaging

Anatomical Sites and Subsites

Lip (C00)
1. External upper lip (vermilion border) (C00.0)
2. External lower lip (vermilion border) (C00.1)
3. Commissures (C00.6)

Oral Cavity (CO2–006)
1. Buccal mucosa
   a) Mucosa of upper and lower lips (C00.3, 4)
   b) Cheek mucosa (C06.0)
   c) Retromolar areas (C06.2)
   d) Buccoalveolar sulci, upper and lower (vestibule of mouth) (C06.1)
2. Upper alveolus and gingiva (upper gum) (C03.0)
3. Lower alveolus and gingiva (lower gum) (C03.14.
4. Hard palate (C05.0)
5. Tongue
   a) Dorsal surface and lateral borders anterior to vallate papillae (anterior two-thirds) (C02.0, 1)
   b) Inferior (ventral) surface (C02.2)
6. Floor of mouth (C04)

Regional Lymph Nodes

The regional lymph nodes are the cervical nodes.

TNM Clinical Classification

T – Primary Tumour

TX   Primary tumour cannot be assessed
T0   No evidence of primary tumour
Tis Carcinoma in situ

T1   Tumour 2 cm or less in greatest dimension and 5 mm or less depth of invasion*

T2   Tumour 2 cm or less in greatest dimension and more than 5 mm but no more than 10 mm depth of invasion or Tumour more than 2 cm but not more than 4 cm in greatest dimension and depth of invasion no more than 10 mm

T3   Tumour more than 4 cm in greatest dimension or more than 10 mm depth of invasion

T4a (Lip) Tumour invades through cortical bone, inferior alveolar nerve, floor of mouth, or skin (of the chin or the nose)

T4a (Oral cavity) Tumour invades through the cortical bone of the mandible or maxillary sinus, or invades the skin of the face

T4b (Lip and oral cavity) Tumour invades masticator space, pterygoid plates, or skull base, or encases internal carotid artery

Note
* Superficial erosion alone of bone/tooth socket by gingival primary is not sufficient to classify a tumour as T4a.

N – Regional Lymph Nodes

NX   Regional lymph nodes cannot be assessed
N0   No regional lymph node metastasis
N1   Metastasis in a single ipsilateral lymph node, 3 cm or less in greatest dimension without extranodal extension
N2   Metastasis described as:
    N2a   Metastasis in a single ipsilateral lymph node, more than 3 cm but not more than 6 cm in greatest dimension without extranodal extension
    N2b   Metastasis in multiple ipsilateral lymph nodes, none more than 6 cm in greatest dimension, without extranodal extension
    N2c   Metastasis in bilateral or contralateral lymph nodes, none more than 6 cm in greatest dimension, without extranodal extension
N3a Metastasis in a lymph node more than 6 cm in greatest dimension without extranodal extension

Head & Neck

N3b   Metastasis in a single or multiple lymph nodes with clinical extranodal extension*

Notes

* The presence of skin involvement or soft tissue invasion with deep fixation/tethering to underlying muscle or adjacent structures or clinical signs of nerve involvement is classified as clinical extranodal extension.

Midline nodes are considered ipsilateral nodes.

M – Distant Metastasis

M0   No distant metastasis
M1   Distant metastasis

pTNM Pathological Classification

The pT categories correspond to the clinical T categories. For pM see page 8.

pN – Regional Lymph Nodes

Histological examination of a selective neck dissection specimen will ordinarily include 10 or more lymph nodes. Histological examination of a radical or modified radical neck dissection specimen will ordinarily include 15 or more lymph nodes.

pNX   Regional lymph nodes cannot be assessed
pN0   No regional lymph node metastasis
pN1   Metastasis in a single ipsilateral lymph node, 3 cm or less in greatest dimension without extranodal extension
pN2   Metastasis described as:
     pN2a   Metastasis in a single ipsilateral lymph node, less than 3 cm in greatest dimension with extranodal extension or, more than 3 cm but not more than 6 cm in greatest dimension without extranodal extension
     pN2b   Metastasis in multiple ipsilateral lymph nodes, none more than 6 cm in greatest dimension, without extranodal extension
     pN2c   Metastasis in bilateral or contralateral lymph nodes, none more than 6 cm in greatest dimension, without extranodal extension
pN3a   Metastasis in a lymph node more than 6 cm in greatest dimension without extranodal extension

pN3b   Metastasis in a lymph node more than 3 cm in greatest dimension with extranodal extension or, multiple ipsilateral, or any contralateral or bilateral node(s) with extranodal extension

Stage

Stage 0	Tis	N0	M0
Stage I	T1	N0	M0
Stage II	T2	N0	M0
Stage III	T3	N0	M0
	T1, T2, T3	N1	M0
Stage IVA	T4a	N0, N1	M0
	T1, T2, T3, T4a	N2	M0
Stage IVB	Any T	N3	M0
	T4b	Any N	M0
Stage IVC	Any T	Any N	M1

Head & Neck

Prognostic Factors Grid – Oral Cavity

Prognostic factors for carcinoma of the oral cavity

Prognostic factors	Tumour related	Host related	Environment related
Essential	T category N category Extracapsular extension (ECE) Surgical resection margin	Performance status Addictions (tobacco/areca nut/alcohol)	Dose of radiotherapy/chemoradiotherapy
Additional	Tumour volume Hypoxia	Age Co-morbidity	Overall treatment/radiation treatment time Interval from surgery to start of postoperative radiotherapy
New and promising	EGFR expression TP53 mutation Bcl-2 ERCC1	Swallowing-related quality of life Global quality of life	

Source: UICC Manual of Clinical Oncology, Ninth Edition. Edited by Brian O'Sullivan, James D. Brierley, Anil K. D'Cruz, Martin F. Fey, Raphael Pollock, Jan B. Vermorken and Shao Hui Huang. © 2015 UICC. Published 2015 by John Wiley & Sons, Ltd.

Pharynx
(ICD-O-3 C01, C05.1-2, C09, C10.0, 2-3, C11-13)

Rules for Classification

The classification applies only to carcinomas. There should be histological confirmation of the disease.

Changes to the seventh edition for carcinoma of the nasopharynx and the introduction of a separate classification for p16-positive oropharyngeal cancer are based on the recommendations referenced.[1,2]

The following are the procedures for assessing T, N, and M categories:

T categories	Physical examination, endoscopy and imaging
N categories	Physical examination and imaging
M categories	Physical examination and imaging

Anatomical Sites and Subsites

Oropharynx (ICD-O-3 C01, C05.1-2, C09.0-1, 9, C10.0, 2-3)

1. Anterior wall (glossoepiglottic area)
   a) Base of tongue (posterior to the vallate papillae or posterior third) (C01)
   b) Vallecula (C10.0)
2. Lateral wall (C 10.2)
   a) Tonsil (C09.9)
   b) Tonsillar fossa (C09.0) and tonsillar (faucial) pillars (C09.1)
   c) Glossotonsillar sulci (tonsillar pillars) (C09.1)
3. Posterior wall (C10.3)
4. Superior wall
   a) Inferior surface of soft palate (C05.1)
   b) Uvula (C05.2)

Nasopharynx (C11)

1. Posterosuperior wall: extends from the level of the junction of the hard and soft palates to the base of the skull (C11.0, 1)
2. Lateral wall: including the fossa of Rosenmüller (C11.2)
3. Inferior wall: consists of the superior surface of the soft palate (C11.3)

Note

The margin of the choanal orifices, including the posterior margin of the nasal septum, is included with the nasal fossa.

Hypopharynx (C12, C13)

1. Pharyngo-oesophageal junction (postcricoid area) (C 13.0): extends from the level of the arytenoid cartilages and connecting folds to the inferior border of the cricoid cartilage, thus forming the anterior wall of the hypopharynx
2. Piriform sinus (C12.9): extends from the pharyngoepiglottic fold to the upper end of the oesophagus. It is bounded laterally by the thyroid cartilage and medially by the hypopharyngeal surface of the aryepiglottic fold (C13.1) and the arytenoid and cricoid cartilages
3. Posterior pharyngeal wall (C 13.2): extends from the superior level of the hyoid bone (or floor of the vallecula) to the level of the inferior border of the cricoid cartilage and from the apex of one piriform sinus to the other

Regional Lymph Nodes

The regional lymph nodes are the cervical nodes.

TNM Clinical Classification

T – Primary Tumour

TX   Primary tumour cannot be assessed
T0   No evidence of primary tumour
Tis   Carcinoma in situ

Oropharynx

p16-negative cancers of the oropharynx or oropharyngeal cancers without a p16 immunohistochemistry performed.

T1   Tumour 2 cm or less in greatest dimension
T2   Tumour more than 2 cm but not more than 4 cm in greatest dimension
T3   Tumour more than 4 cm in greatest dimension or extension to lingual surface of epiglottis
T4a   Tumour invades any of the following: larynx,* deep/extrinsic muscle of tongue (genioglossus, hyoglossus, palatoglossus, and styloglossus), medial pterygoid, hard palate, or mandible
T4b   Tumour invades any of the following: lateral pterygoid muscle, pterygoid plates, lateral nasopharynx, skull base; or encases carotid artery

Head & Neck

Note

* Mucosal extension to lingual surface of epiglottis from primary tumours of the base of the tongue and vallecula does not constitute invasion of the larynx.

Oropharynx – p16-Positive Tumours

Tumours that have positive p16 immunohistochemistry overexpression.

T1   Tumour 2 cm or less in greatest dimension

T2   Tumour more than 2 cm but not more than 4 cm in greatest dimension

T3   Tumour more than 4 cm in greatest dimension or extension to lingual surface of epiglottis

T4   Tumour invades any of the following: larynx*, deep/extrinsic muscle of tongue (genioglossus, hyoglossus, palatoglossus, and styloglossus), medial pterygoid, hard palate, mandible*, lateral pterygoid muscle, pterygoid plates, lateral nasopharynx, skull base; or encases carotid artery

Note

* Mucosal extension to lingual surface of epiglottis from primary tumours of the base of the tongue and vallecula does not constitute invasion of the larynx.

Hypopharynx

T1   Tumour limited to one subsite of hypopharynx (see page 23 and/or 2 cm or less in greatest dimension

T2   Tumour invades more than one subsite of hypopharynx or an adjacent site, or measures more than 2 cm but not more than 4 cm in greatest dimension, without fixation of hemilarynx

T3   Tumour more than 4 cm in greatest dimension, or with fixation of hemilarynx or extension to oesophagus

T4a   Tumour invades any of the following: thyroid/cricoid cartilage, hyoid bone, thyroid gland, oesophagus, central compartment soft tissue*

T4b   Tumour invades prevertebral fascia, encases carotid artery, or invades mediastinal structures

Note

* Central compartment soft tissue includes prelaryngeal strap muscles and subcutaneous fat.

Nasopharynx

T1   Tumour confined to nasopharynx, or extends to oropharynx and/or nasal cavity without parapharyngeal involvement

T2   Tumour with extension to parapharyngeal space and/or infiltration of the medial pterygoid, lateral pterygoid, and/or prevertebral muscles

T3   Tumour invades bony structures of skull base cervical vertebra, pterygoid structures, and/or paranasal sinuses

T4   Tumour with intracranial extension and/or involvement of cranial nerves, hypopharynx, orbit, parotid gland and/or infiltration beyond the lateral surface of the lateral pterygoid muscle

N – Regional Lymph Nodes

Oropharynx – p16-Negative and Hypopharynx

NX   Regional lymph nodes cannot be assessed

N0   No regional lymph node metastasis

N1   Metastasis in a single ipsilateral lymph node, 3 cm or less in greatest dimension without extranodal extension

N2   Metastasis described as:

     N2a   Metastasis in a single ipsilateral lymph node more than 3 cm but not more than 6 cm in greatest dimension without extranodal extension

     N2b   Metastasis in multiple ipsilateral lymph nodes, none more than 6 cm in greatest dimension, without extranodal extension

     N2c   Metastasis in bilateral or contralateral lymph nodes, none more than 6 cm in greatest dimension, without extranodal extension

N3a   Metastasis in a lymph node more than 6 cm in greatest dimension without extranodal extension

N3b   Metastasis in a single or multiple lymph nodes with clinical extranodal extension*

Notes

* The presence of skin involvement or soft tissue invasion with deep fixation/tethering to underlying muscle or adjacent structures or clinical signs of nerve involvement is classified as clinical extranodal extension.

Midline nodes are considered ipsilateral nodes.

Oropharynx p-16 Positive
Clinical

NX   Regional lymph nodes cannot be assessed

N0   No regional lymph node metastasis

N1   Unilateral metastasis, in lymph node(s), all 6 cm or less in greatest dimension

N2   Contralateral or bilateral metastasis in lymph node(s), all 6 cm or less in greatest dimension

N3   Metastasis in lymph node(s) greater than 6 cm in dimension

Note
Midline nodes are considered ipsilateral nodes.

Nasopharynx

NX   Regional lymph nodes cannot be assessed

N0   No regional lymph node metastasis

N1   Unilateral metastasis, in cervical lymph node(s), and/or unilateral or bilateral metastasis in retropharyngeal lymph nodes, 6 cm or less in greatest dimension, above the caudal border of cricoid cartilage

N2   Bilateral metastasis in cervical lymph node(s), 6 cm or less in greatest dimension, above the caudal border of cricoid cartilage

N3   Metastasis in cervical lymph node(s) greater than 6 cm in dimension and/or extension below the caudal border of cricoid cartilage

Note
Midline nodes are considered ipsilateral nodes.

M – Distant Metastasis

M0   No distant metastasis

M1   Distant metastasis

pTNM Pathological Classification

The pT categories correspond to the T categories. For pM see page 8.

Histological examination of a selective neck dissection specimen will ordinarily include 10 or more lymph nodes. Histological examination of a radical or modified radical neck dissection specimen will ordinarily include 15 or more lymph nodes.

Oropharynx – p16 Negative and Hypopharynx

pNX   Regional lymph nodes cannot be assessed

pN0   No regional lymph node metastasis

pN1   Metastasis in a single ipsilateral lymph node, 3 cm or less in greatest dimension without extranodal extension

pN2   Metastasis described as:

pN2a   Metastasis in a single ipsilateral lymph node, less than 3 cm in greatest dimension with extranodal extension or more than 3 cm but not more than 6 cm in greatest dimension without extranodal extension

pN2b   Metastasis in multiple ipsilateral lymph nodes, none more than 6 cm in greatest dimension, without extranodal extension

pN2c   Metastasis in bilateral or contralateral lymph nodes, none more than 6 cm in greatest dimension, without extranodal extension

pN3a   Metastasis in a lymph node more than 6 cm in greatest dimension without extranodal extension

pN3b   Metastasis in a lymph node more than 3 cm in greatest dimension with extranodal extension or, multiple ipsilateral, or any contralateral or bilateral node(s) with extranodal extension

Oropharynx p-16 Positive

pNX   Regional lymph nodes cannot be assessed
pN0   No regional lymph node metastasis
pN1   Metastasis in 1 to 4 lymph node(s)
pN2   Metastasis in 5 or more lymph node(s)

Nasopharynx

The pN categories correspond to the N categories

Stage (Oropharynx – p16 Negative and Hypopharynx)

Stage 0	Tis	N0	M0
Stage I	T1	N0	M0
Stage II	T2	N0	M0
Stage III	T3	N0	M0
	T1, T2, T3	N1	M0
Stage IVA	T1, T2, T3	N2	M0
	T4a	N0, N1, N2	M0
Stage IVB	T4b	Any N	M0
	Any T	N3	M0
Stage IVC	Any T	Any N	M1

Head & Neck

Stage (Oropharynx –p16 Positive)

Clinical

Stage 0	Tis	N0	M0
Stage I	T1, T2	N0, N1	M0
Stage II	T1, T2	N2	M0
	T3	N0, N1, N2	M0
Stage III	T1, T2, T3	N3	M0
	T4	Any	M0
Stage IV	Any T	Any N	M1

Pathological

Stage 0	Tis	N0	M0
Stage I	T1, T2	N0, 1	M0
Stage II	T1, T2	N2	M0
	T3	N0, N1	M0
Stage III	T3, T4	N2	M0
Stage IV	Any T	Any N	M1

Stage (Nasopharynx)

Stage 0	Tis	N0	M0
Stage I	T1	N0	M0
Stage II	T1	N1	M0
	T2	N0, N1	M0
Stage III	T1, T2	N2	M0
	T3	N0, N1, N2	M0
Stage IVA	T4	N0, N1, N2	M0
Stage IVA	Any T	N3	M0
Stage IVB	Any T	Any N	M1

Prognostic Factors Grid

Oropharynx

Prognostic risk factors for survival of OPC

Prognostic factors	Tumour related	Host related	Environment related
Essential	HPV status (including p16) T category N category	Smoking, especially during radiotherapy Performance status	Quality of treating facility (staging workup and expertise in multidisciplinary management)
Additional	Number of involved nodes Level of involved nodes Tumour volume Hypoxia	Co-morbidities Age	Ability to receive standard treatment: ▪ Radiation dose ▪ Overall treatment time ▪ Quality of radiotherapy
New and promising	EGFR expression TP53 mutation Bcl-2 ERCC1	Health-related quality of life	

Source: UICC Manual of Clinical Oncology, Ninth Edition. Edited by Brian O'Sullivan, James D. Brierley, Anil K. D'Cruz, Martin F. Fey, Raphael Pollock, Jan B. Vermorken and Shao Hui Huang. © 2015 UICC. Published 2015 by John Wiley & Sons, Ltd.

Head & Neck

Nasopharynx

Prognostic factors for nasopharyngeal carcinoma

Prognostic factors	Tumour related	Host related	Environment related
Essential	Presenting stage Histological type	Age Performance status Co-morbidities	Facilities for staging work-up (MRI, PET-CT) Facilities for high-quality radiotherapy (conformal techniques and precision) Appropriate addition of chemotherapy Expertise in radiotherapy and chemotherapy
Additional	EBV-DNA Gross tumour volume Site of metastases	LDH	Optimization of radiotherapy dose fractionation Optimization of chemotherapy sequence and drugs
New and promising	Biomarkers Gene signatures		Advances in diagnostic and therapeutic technology

Source: UICC Manual of Clinical Oncology, Ninth Edition. Edited by Brian O'Sullivan, James D. Brierley, Anil K. D'Cruz, Martin F. Fey, Raphael Pollock, Jan B. Vermorken and Shao Hui Huang. © 2015 UICC. Published 2015 by John Wiley & Sons, Ltd.

References

1 Pan JJ, Ng WT, Zong J F, et al. Proposal for the 8th edition of the AJCC/UICC staging system for nasopharyngeal cancer in the era of intensity-modulated radiotherapy. *Cancer* 2016; 122: 546–558.

2 O'Sullivan B, Huang SH, Su J, et al. A proposal for UICC/AJCC pre-treatment TNM staging for HPV-related oropharyngeal cancer by the International Collaboration on Oropharyngeal Cancer Network for Staging (ICON-S): A comparative multi-centre cohort study. *Lancet Oncol* 2016; 17: 440–451.

Larynx
(ICD-O-3 C32.0-2, C10.1)

Rules for Classification

The classification applies only to carcinomas. There should be histological confirmation of the disease.

The following are the procedures for assessing T, N, and M categories:

T categories   Physical examination, laryngoscopy, and imaging
N categories   Physical examination and imaging
M categories   Physical examination and imaging

Anatomical Sites and Subsites

1. Supraglottis (C32.1)
    a) Suprahyoid epiglottis [including tip, lingual (anterior) (C 10.1), and laryngeal surfaces]   } *Epilarynx (including marginal zone)*
    b) Aryepiglottic fold, laryngeal aspect
    c) Arytenoid
    d) Infrahyoid epiglottis   } *Supraglottis excluding epilarynx*
    e) Ventricular bands (false cords)
2. Glottis (C32.0)
    a) Vocal cords
    b) Anterior commissure
    c) Posterior commissure
3. Subglottis (C32.2)

Regional Lymph Nodes

The regional lymph nodes are the cervical nodes.

TNM Clinical Classification

T – Primary Tumour

TX   Primary tumour cannot be assessed
T0   No evidence of primary tumour
Tis   Carcinoma in situ

Supraglottis

T1 Tumour limited to one subsite of supraglottis with normal vocal cord mobility

T2 Tumour invades mucosa of more than one adjacent subsite of supraglottis or glottis or region outside the supraglottis (e.g., mucosa of base of tongue, vallecula, medial wall of piriform sinus) without fixation of the larynx

T3 Tumour limited to larynx with vocal cord fixation and/or invades any of the following: postcricoid area, pre-epiglottic space, paraglottic space, and/or inner cortex of thyroid cartilage

T4a Tumour invades through the thyroid cartilage and/or invades tissues beyond the larynx, e.g., trachea, soft tissues of neck including deep/extrinsic muscle of tongue (genioglossus, hyoglossus, palatoglossus, and styloglossus), strap muscles, thyroid, or oesophagus

T4b Tumour invades prevertebral space, encases carotid artery, or mediastinal structures

Glottis

T1 Tumour limited to vocal cord(s) (may involve anterior or posterior commissure) with normal mobility

    T1a Tumour limited to one vocal cord

    T1b Tumour involves both vocal cords

T2 Tumour extends to supraglottis and/or subglottis, and/or with impaired vocal cord mobility

T3 Tumour limited to larynx with vocal cord fixation and/or invades paraglottic space, and/or inner cortex of the thyroid cartilage

T4a Tumour invades through the outer cortex of the thyroid cartilage, and/or invades tissues beyond the larynx, e.g., trachea, soft tissues of neck including deep/extrinsic muscle of tongue (genioglossus, hyoglossus, palatoglossus, and styloglossus), strap muscles, thyroid, oesophagus

T4b Tumour invades prevertebral space, encases carotid artery, or mediastinal structures

Subglottis

T1 Tumour limited to subglottis

T2 Tumour extends to vocal cord(s) with normal or impaired mobility

T3 Tumour limited to larynx with vocal cord fixation

T4a Tumour invades cricoid or thyroid cartilage and/or invades tissues beyond the larynx, e.g., trachea, soft tissues of neck including deep/

extrinsic muscle of tongue (genioglossus, hyoglossus, pala toglossus, and styloglossus), strap muscles, thyroid, oesophagus

T4b Tumour invades prevertebral space, encases carotid artery, or mediastinal structures

N – Regional Lymph Nodes

N1 Metastasis in a single ipsilateral lymph node, 3 cm or less in greatest dimension without extranodal extension

N2 Metastasis described as:

N2a Metastasis in a single ipsilateral lymph node, more than 3 cm but not more than 6 cm in greatest dimension without extranodal extension

N2b Metastasis in multiple ipsilateral lymph nodes, none more than 6 cm in greatest dimension, without extranodal extension

N2c Metastasis in bilateral or contralateral lymph nodes, none more than 6 cm in greatest dimension, without extranodal extension

N3a Metastasis in a lymph node more than 6 cm in greatest dimension without extranodal extension

N3b Metastasis in a single or multiple lymph nodes with clinical extranodal extension*

Notes

* The presence of skin involvement or soft tissue invasion with deep fixation/tethering to underlying muscle or adjacent structures or clinical signs of nerve involvement is classified as clinical extra nodal extension.

Midline nodes are considered ipsilateral nodes.

M – Distant Metastasis

M0 No distant metastasis

M1 Distant metastasis

pTNM Pathological Classification

The pT categories correspond to the clinical T categories. For pM see page 8.

pN – Regional Lymph Nodes

Histological examination of a selective neck dissection specimen will ordinarily include 10 or more lymph nodes. Histological examination of a radical or modified radical neck dissection specimen will ordinarily include 15 or more lymph nodes.

pNX	Regional lymph nodes cannot be assessed
pN0	No regional lymph node metastasis
pN1	Metastasis in a single ipsilateral lymph node, 3 cm or less in greatest dimension without extranodal extension
pN2	Metastasis described as:

pN2a   Metastasis in a single ipsilateral lymph node, less than 3 cm in greatest dimension with extranodal extension or more than 3 cm but not more than 6 cm in greatest dimension without extranodal extension

pN2b   Metastasis in multiple ipsilateral lymph nodes, none more than 6 cm in greatest dimension, without extranodal extension

pN2c   Metastasis in bilateral or contralateral lymph nodes, none more than 6 cm in greatest dimension, without extranodal extension

pN3a   Metastasis in a lymph node more than 6 cm in greatest dimension without extranodal extension

pN3b   Metastasis in a lymph node more than 3 cm in greatest dimension with extranodal extension or multiple ipsilateral, or any contralateral or bilateral node(s) with extranodal extension

Stage

Stage 0	Tis	N0	M0
Stage I	T1	N0	M0
Stage II	T2	N0	M0
Stage III	T3	N0	M0
	T1,T2,T3	N1	M0
Stage IVA	T4a	N0, N1	M0
	T1,T2,T3,T4a	N2	M0
Stage IVB	T4b	Any N	M0
	Any T	N3	M0
Stage IVC	Any T	Any N	M1

Prognostic Factors Grid

Prognostic factors for survival for laryngeal and hypopharyngeal carcinoma

Prognostic factors	Tumour related	Host related	Environment related
Essential	T, N, M categories Extracapsular extension	Co-morbidities Age >70 years Performance status	Able to provide standard treatment (resources) Treatment quality Resection margins
Additional	Regions/subsites involved Low neck nodes Tumour volume Vocal cord impairment Tracheostomy	Gender Laryngeal function	Nutrition Social/ environmental (e.g. anatomical station) Overall treatment time
New and promising	Tumour markers: TP53, VEGF, cyclin D1 amplifi cation, EGFR, Bcl-2 Tumour HPV status Chemoresistance genes	Baseline quality of life	Optical imaging New sensitizers in photodynamic therapy

Source: UICC Manual of Clinical Oncology, Ninth Edition. Edited by Brian O'Sullivan, James D. Brierley, Anil K. D'Cruz, Martin F. Fey, Raphael Pollock, Jan B. Vermorken and Shao Hui Huang. © 2015 UICC. Published 2015 by John Wiley & Sons, Ltd.

Head & Neck

Nasal Cavity and Paranasal Sinuses (ICD-O-3 C30.0, 31.0-1)

Rules for Classification

The classification applies only to carcinomas. There should be histological confirmation of the disease.

The following are the procedures for assessing T, N, and M categories:

T *categories*   Physical examination and imaging
N *categories*   Physical examination and imaging
M *categories*   Physical examination and imaging

Anatomical Sites and Subsites

1. Nasal cavity (C30.0)
   - Septum
   - Floor
   - Lateral wall
   - Vestibule
2. Maxillary sinus (C31.0)
3. Ethmoid sinus (C31.1)
   - Left
   - Right

Regional Lymph Nodes

The regional lymph nodes are the cervical nodes.

TNM Clinical Classification

T – Primary Tumour

TX   Primary tumour cannot be assessed
T0   No evidence of primary tumour
Tis   Carcinoma in situ

Maxillary Sinus

T1   Tumour limited to the mucosa with no erosion or destruction of bone
T2   Tumour causing bone erosion or destruction, including extension into the hard palate and/or middle nasal meatus, except extension to posterior wall of maxillary sinus and pterygoid plates

T3   Tumour invades any of the following: bone of posterior wall of maxillary sinus, subcutaneous tissues, floor or medial wall of orbit, pterygoid fossa, or ethmoid sinuses

T4a   Tumour invades any of the following: anterior orbital contents, skin of cheek, pterygoid plates, infratemporal fossa, cribriform plate, sphenoid or frontal sinuses

T4b   Tumour invades any of the following: orbital apex, dura, brain, middle cranial fossa, cranial nerves other than maxillary division of trigeminal nerve (V2), nasopharynx, or clivus

Nasal Cavity and Ethmoid Sinus

T1   Tumour restricted to one subsite of nasal cavity or ethmoid sinus, with or without bony invasion

T2   Tumour involves two subsites in a single site or extends to involve an adjacent site within the nasoethmoidal complex, with or without bony invasion

T3   Tumour extends to invade the medial wall or floor of the orbit, maxillary sinus, palate, or cribriform plate

T4a   Tumour invades any of the following: anterior orbital contents, skin of nose or cheek, minimal extension to anterior cranial fossa, pterygoid plates, sphenoid or frontal sinuses

T4b   Tumour invades any of the following: orbital apex, dura, brain, middle cranial fossa, cranial nerves other than V2, nasopharynx, or clivus

N – Regional Lymph Nodes

N1   Metastasis in a single ipsilateral lymph node, 3 cm or less in greatest dimension without extranodal extension

N2   Metastasis described as:

    N2a   Metastasis in a single ipsilateral lymph node, more than 3 cm but not more than 6 cm in greatest dimension without extranodal extension

    N2b   Metastasis in multiple ipsilateral lymph nodes, none more than 6 cm in greatest dimension, without extranodal extension

    N2c   Metastasis in bilateral or contralateral lymph nodes, none more than 6 cm in greatest dimension, without extranodal extension

N3a   Metastasis in a lymph node more than 6 cm in greatest dimension without extranodal extension

N3b   Metastasis in a single or multiple lymph nodes with clinical extranodal extension*

Head & Neck

Notes

* The presence of skin involvement or soft tissue invasion with deep fixation/ tethering to underlying muscle or adjacent structures or clinical signs of nerve involvement is classified as clinical extra nodal extension.

Midline nodes are considered ipsilateral nodes.

M – Distant Metastasis

M0   No distant metastasis

M1   Distant metastasis

pTNM Pathological Classification

The pT categories correspond to the clinical T categories. For pM see page 8.

pN – Regional Lymph Nodes

Histological examination of a selective neck dissection specimen will ordinarily include 10 or more lymph nodes. Histological examination of a radical or modified radical neck dissection specimen will ordinarily include 15 or more lymph nodes.

pNX   Regional lymph nodes cannot be assessed

pN0   No regional lymph node metastasis

pN1   Metastasis in a single ipsilateral lymph node, 3 cm or less in greatest dimension without extranodal extension

pN2   Metastasis described as:

   pN2a   Metastasis in a single ipsilateral lymph node, less than 3 cm in greatest dimension with extranodal extension or, more than 3 cm but not more than 6 cm in greatest dimension without extranodal extension

   pN2b   Metastasis in multiple ipsilateral lymph nodes, none more than 6 cm in greatest dimension, without extranodal extension

   pN2c   Metastasis in bilateral or contralateral lymph nodes, none more than 6 cm in greatest dimension, without extranodal extension

pN3a   Metastasis in a lymph node more than 6 cm in greatest dimension without extranodal extension

pN3b   Metastasis in a lymph node more than 3 cm in greatest dimension with extranodal extension or multiple ipsilateral, or any contralateral or bilateral node(s) with extranodal extension

Stage

Stage 0	Tis	N0	M0
Stage I	T1	N0	M0
Stage II	T2	N0	M0
Stage III	T3	N0	M0
	T1, T2, T3	N1	M0
Stage IVA	T1, T2, T3	N2	M0
	T4a	N0, N1, N2	M0
Stage IVB	T4b	Any N	M0
	Any T	N3	M0
Stage IVC	Any T	Any N	M1

Prognostic Factors Grid – Nasal Cavity and Paranasal Sinuses

Prognostic factors for paranasal sinus tumours

Prognostic factors	Tumour related	Host related	Environment related
Essential	T category N category M category		
Additional	Histotype	Age Gender Performance status	Radiation dose Overall treatment time Surgical margins
New and promising			High precision optimal dose radiation Concurrent cytotoxic or biological therapies Ideal integration with advanced surgical techniques

Source: UICC Manual of Clinical Oncology, Ninth Edition. Edited by Brian O'Sullivan, James D. Brierley, Anil K. D'Cruz, Martin F. Fey, Raphael Pollock, Jan B. Vermorken and Shao Hui Huang. © 2015 UICC. Published 2015 by John Wiley & Sons, Ltd.

Unknown Primary – Cervical Nodes

Rules for Classification

There should be histological confirmation of squamous cell carcinoma with lymph node metastases but without an identified primary carcinoma. Histological methods should be used to identify EBV and HPV/p16-related tumours. If there is evidence of EBV, the nasopharyngeal classification is applied. If there is evidence of HPV and positive immunohistochemistry p16 overexpression, the p16-positive oropharyngeal classification is applied.

TNM Clinical Classification

EBV or HPV/p16 negative or unknown

T – Primary Tumour

T0   No evidence of primary tumour

N – Regional Lymph Nodes

N1   Metastasis in a single ipsilateral lymph node, 3 cm or less in greatest dimension without extranodal extension

N2   Metastasis described as:

    N2a   Metastasis in a single ipsilateral lymph node, more than 3 cm but not more than 6 cm in greatest dimension without extranodal extension

    N2b   Metastasis in multiple ipsilateral lymph nodes, none more than 6 cm in greatest dimension, without extranodal extension

    N2c   Metastasis in bilateral or contralateral lymph nodes, none more than 6 cm in greatest dimension, without extranodal extension

N3a   Metastasis in a lymph node more than 6 cm in greatest dimension without extranodal extension

N3b   Metastasis in a single or multiple lymph nodes with clinical extranodal extension*

Notes
* The presence of skin involvement or soft tissue invasion with deep fixation/ tethering to underlying muscle or adjacent structures or clinical signs of nerve involvement is classified as clinical extra nodal extension.
Midline nodes are considered ipsilateral nodes.

M – Distant Metastasis

M0   No distant metastasis
M1   Distant metastasis

pTNM Pathological Classification

The pT category corresponds to the clinical T category.
For pM see page 8.

pN – Regional Lymph Nodes

Histological examination of a selective neck dissection specimen will ordinarily include 10 or more lymph nodes. Histological examination of a radical or modified radical neck dissection specimen will ordinarily include 15 or more lymph nodes.

pN1   Metastasis in a single ipsilateral lymph node, 3 cm or less in greatest dimension without extranodal extension

pN2   Metastasis described as:

pN2a   Metastasis in a single ipsilateral lymph node, less than 3 cm in greatest dimension with extranodal extension or more than 3 cm but not more than 6 cm in greatest dimension without extranodal extension

pN2b   Metastasis in multiple ipsilateral lymph nodes, none more than 6 cm in greatest dimension, without extranodal extension

pN2c   Metastasis in bilateral or contralateral lymph nodes, none more than 6 cm in greatest dimension, without extranodal extension

pN3a   Metastasis in a lymph node more than 6 cm in greatest dimension without extranodal extension

pN3b   Metastasis in a lymph node more than 3 cm in greatest dimension with extranodal extension or multiple ipsilateral, or any contralateral, or bilateral node(s) with extranodal extension

Stage

Stage III	T0	N1	M0
Stage IVA	T0	N2	M0
Stage IVB	T0	N3	M0
Stage IVC	T0	N1, N2, N3	M1

Head & Neck

TNM Clinical Classification

HPV/p16 positive

T – Primary Tumour

T0   No evidence of primary tumour

N – Regional Lymph Nodes

N1   Unilateral metastasis, in cervical lymph node(s), all 6 cm or less in greatest dimension
N2   Contralateral or bilateral metastasis in cervical lymph node(s), all 6 cm or less in greatest dimension
N3   Metastasis in cervical lymph node(s) greater than 6 cm in dimension

pTNM Pathological Classification

There is no pT category.

pN – Regional Lymph Nodes

Histological examination of a selective neck dissection specimen will ordinarily include 10 or more lymph nodes. Histological examination of a radical or modified radical neck dissection specimen will ordinarily include 15 or more lymph nodes.

pN1   Metastasis in 1 to 4 lymph node(s)
pN2   Metastasis in 5 or more lymph node(s)

Stage

Clinical

Stage			
Stage I	T0	N1	M0
Stage II	T0	N2	M0
Stage III	T0	N3	M0
Stage IV	T0	N1, N2, N3	M1

Pathological

Stage			
Stage I	T0	N1	M0
Stage II	T0	N2	M0
Stage IV	T0	N1, N2	M1

TNM Clinical Classification

EBV positive

T – Primary Tumour

T0   No evidence of primary tumour

N – Regional Lymph Nodes *(Nasopharynx)*

N1   Unilateral metastasis, in cervical lymph node(s), and/or unilateral or bilateral metastasis in retropharyngeal lymph nodes, 6 cm or less in greatest dimension, above the caudal border of cricoid cartilage

N2   Bilateral metastasis in cervical lymph node(s), 6 cm or less in greatest dimension, above the caudal border of cricoid cartilage

N3   Metastasis in cervical lymph node(s) greater than 6 cm in dimension and/or extension below the caudal border of cricoid cartilage

Note
Midline nodes are considered ipsilateral nodes.

pTNM Pathological Classification

The pT and pN categories correspond to the T and N categories. For pM see page 8.

pN0   Histological examination of a selective neck dissection specimen will ordinarily include 10 or more lymph nodes. Histological examination of a radical or modified radical neck dissection specimen will ordinarily include 15 or more lymph nodes.

M – Distant Metastasis

M0   No distant metastasis

Stage

Stage II	T0	N1	M0
Stage III	T0	N2	M0
Stage IVA	T0	N3	M0
Stage IVB	T0	N1, N2, N3	M1

Head & Neck

Prognostic Factors Grid – Cervical Nodes Unknown Primary

Prognostic factors for head and neck unknown primary

Prognostic factors	Tumour related	Host related	Environment related
Essential	Histology N category and number of nodes Extracapsular extension Presence or absence of metastatic disease p16^{INK4A}/HPV status, or EBV DNA status	Immunosuppression (especially skin cancer)	
Additional	Tumour differentiation Location of nodal disease (above vs below clavicle)	Gender Haemoglobin level Smoking history	Subsequent discovery of primary Overall treatment time
New and Promising	TP53 Surviving nuclear expression		

Source: UICC Manual of Clinical Oncology, Ninth Edition. Edited by Brian O'Sullivan, James D. Brierley, Anil K. D'Cruz, Martin F. Fey, Raphael Pollock, Jan B. Vermorken and Shao Hui Huang. © 2015 UICC. Published 2015 by John Wiley & Sons, Ltd.

Malignant Melanoma of Upper Aerodigestive Tract
(ICD-O-3 C00-06, 10-14, 30-32)

Rules for Classification

The classification applies only to mucosal malignant melanomas of the head and neck region, i.e., of the upper aerodigestive tract. There should be histological confirmation of the disease and division of cases by site.

The following are the procedures for assessing T, N, and M categories:

T *categories*	Physical examination and imaging
N *categories*	Physical examination and imaging
M *categories*	Physical examination and imaging

Regional Lymph Nodes

The regional lymph nodes are those appropriate to the site of the primary tumour. See page 17.

TNM Clinical Classification

T – Primary Tumour

TX	Primary tumour cannot be assessed
T0	No evidence of primary tumour
T3	Tumour limited to the epithelium and/or submucosa (mucosal disease)
T4a	Tumour invades deep soft tissue, cartilage, bone, or overlying skin
T4b	Tumour invades any of the following: brain, dura, skull base, lower cranial nerves (IX, X, XI, XII), masticator space, carotid artery, prevertebral space, mediastinal structures

Note

Mucosal melanomas are aggressive tumours, therefore T1 and T2 are omitted as are stages I and II.

N – Regional Lymph Nodes

NX	Regional lymph nodes cannot be assessed
N0	No regional lymph node metastasis
N1	Regional lymph node metastasis

Head & Neck

M – Distant Metastasis

M0 No distant metastasis
M1 Distant metastasis

pTNM Pathological Classification

The pT and pN categories correspond to the T and N categories. For pM see page 8.

pN0 Histological examination of a regional lymphadenectomy specimen will ordinarily include 6 or more lymph nodes. If the lymph nodes are negative, but the number ordinarily examined is not met, classify as pN0.

Stage

Stage III	T3	N0	M0
Stage IVA	T4a	N0	M0
	T3, T4a	N1	M0
Stage IVB	T4b	Any N	M0
Stage IVC	Any T	Any N	M1

Major Salivary Glands
(ICD-O-3 C07, C08)

Rules for Classification

The classification applies only to carcinomas of the major salivary glands. Tumours arising in minor salivary glands (mucus-secreting glands in the lining membrane of the upper aerodigestive tract) are not included in this classification but at their anatomic site of origin, e.g., lip. There should be histological confirmation of the disease.

The following are the procedures for assessing T, N, and M categories:

T *categories*	Physical examination and imaging
N *categories*	Physical examination and imaging
M *categories*	Physical examination and imaging

Anatomical Sites

- Parotid gland (C07.9)
- Submandibular (submaxillary) gland (C08.0)
- Sublingual gland (C08.1)

Regional Lymph Nodes

The regional lymph nodes are the cervical nodes.

TNM Clinical Classification

T – Primary Tumour

TX	Primary tumour cannot be assessed
T0	No evidence of primary tumour
T1	Tumour 2 cm or less in greatest dimension without extraparenchymal extension*
T2	Tumour more than 2 cm but not more than 4 cm in greatest dimension without extraparenchymal extension*
T3	Tumour more than 4 cm and/or tumour with extraparenchymal extension*
T4a	Tumour invades skin, mandible, ear canal, and/or facial nerve
T4b	Tumour invades base of skull, and/or pterygoid plates, and/or encases carotid artery

Note
* Extraparenchymal extension is clinical or macroscopic evidence of invasion of soft tissues or nerve, except those listed under T4a and T4b. Microscopic evidence alone does not constitute extraparenchymal extension for classification purposes.

N – Regional Lymph Nodes

N1   Metastasis in a single ipsilateral lymph node, 3 cm or less in greatest dimension without extranodal extension

N2   Metastasis described as:

      N2a   Metastasis in a single ipsilateral lymph node, more than 3 cm but not more than 6 cm in greatest dimension without extranodal extension

      N2b   Metastasis in multiple ipsilateral lymph nodes, none more than 6 cm in greatest dimension, without extranodal extension

      N2c   Metastasis in bilateral or contralateral lymph nodes, none more than 6 cm in greatest dimension, without extranodal extension

N3a   Metastasis in a lymph node more than 6 cm in greatest dimension without extranodal extension

N3b   Metastasis in a single or multiple lymph nodes with clinical extranodal extension*

Notes
* The presence of skin involvement or soft tissue invasion with deep fixation/tethering to underlying muscle or adjacent structures or clinical signs of nerve involvement is classified as clinical extra nodal extension.
Midline nodes are considered ipsilateral nodes.

M – Distant Metastasis

M0   No distant metastasis
M1   Distant metastasis

pTNM Pathological Classification

The pT categories correspond to the clinical T categories. For pM see page 8.

pN – Regional Lymph Nodes

Histological examination of a selective neck dissection specimen will ordinarily include 10 or more lymph nodes. Histological examination of a radical or modified radical neck dissection specimen will ordinarily include 15 or more lymph nodes.

pNX	Regional lymph nodes cannot be assessed
pN0	No regional lymph node metastasis
pN1	Metastasis in a single ipsilateral lymph node, 3 cm or less in greatest dimension without extranodal extension
pN2	Metastasis described as:

pN2a   Metastasis in a single ipsilateral lymph node, less than 3 cm in greatest dimension with extranodal extension or, more than 3 cm but not more than 6 cm in greatest dimension without extranodal extension

pN2b   Metastasis in multiple ipsilateral lymph nodes, none more than 6 cm in greatest dimension, without extranodal extension

pN2c   Metastasis in bilateral or contralateral lymph nodes, none more than 6 cm in greatest dimension, without extranodal extension

pN3a   Metastasis in a lymph node more than 6 cm in greatest dimension without extranodal extension

pN3b   Metastasis in a lymph node more than 3 cm in greatest dimension with extranodal extension or multiple ipsilateral, or any contralateral, or bilateral node(s) with extranodal extension

Head & Neck

Stage

Stage 0	Tis	N0	M0
Stage I	T1	N0	M0
Stage II	T2	N0	M0
Stage III	T3	N0	M0
	T1, T2, T3	N1	M0
Stage IVA	T1, T2, T3,	N2	M0
	T4a	N0, N1, N2	M0
Stage IVB	T4b	Any N	M0
	Any T	N3	M0
Stage IVC	Any T	Any N	M1

Prognostic Factors Grid – Major Salivary Glands

Prognostic factors for salivary gland tumour survival

Prognostic factors	Tumour related	Host related	Environment related
Essential	Histological grade Tumour size Local invasion Perineural invasion	Age	Resection margins and residual disease (R0/R1/R2)
Additional	Nodal metastases	Facial palsy, pain	Adjuvant radiotherapy
New and promising	Molecular markers (c-Kit, Ki-67, HER2, EGFR, VEGF, androgen receptors)		Neutron vs photon radiotherapy

Source: UICC Manual of Clinical Oncology, Ninth Edition. Edited by Brian O'Sullivan, James D. Brierley, Anil K. D'Cruz, Martin F. Fey, Raphael Pollock, Jan B. Vermorken and Shao Hui Huang. © 2015 UICC. Published 2015 by John Wiley & Sons, Ltd.

Thyroid Gland
(ICD-O-3 C73.9)

Rules for Classification

The classification applies only to carcinomas. There should be microscopic confirmation of the disease and division of cases by histological type.

The following are the procedures for assessing T, N, and M categories:

T categories   Physical examination, endoscopy, and imaging
N categories   Physical examination and imaging
M categories   Physical examination and imaging

Regional Lymph Nodes

The regional lymph nodes are the cervical and upper/superior mediastinal nodes.

TNM Clinical Classification

T – Primary Tumour*

TX   Primary tumour cannot be assessed
T0   No evidence of primary tumour

T1   Tumour 2 cm or less in greatest dimension, limited to the thyroid
     T1a   Tumour 1 cm or less in greatest dimension, limited to the thyroid
     T1b   Tumour more than 1 cm but not more than 2 cm in greatest dimension, limited to the thyroid
T2   Tumour more than 2 cm but not more than 4 cm in greatest dimension, limited to the thyroid
T3   Tumour more than 4 cm in greatest dimension, limited to the thyroid or with gross extrathyroidal extension invading only strap muscles (sternohyoid, sternothyroid, or omohyoid muscles)
     T3a   Tumour more than 4 cm in greatest dimension, limited to the thyroid
     T3b   Tumour of any size with gross extrathyroidal extension invading strap muscles (sternohyoid, sternothyroid, or omohyoid muscles)
T4a   Tumour extends beyond the thyroid capsule and invades any of the following: subcutaneous soft tissues, larynx, trachea, oesophagus, recurrent laryngeal nerve

Head & Neck

T4b Tumour invades prevertebral fascia, mediastinal vessels, or encases carotid artery

Note

* Including papillary, follicular, poorly differentiated, Hurthle cell and anaplastic carcinomas.

N – Regional Lymph Nodes

NX Regional lymph nodes cannot be assessed
N0 No regional lymph node metastasis
N1 Regional lymph node metastasis
  N1a Metastasis in Level VI (pretracheal, paratracheal, and prelaryngeal/Delphian lymph nodes) or upper/superior mediastinum
  N1b Metastasis in other unilateral, bilateral or contralateral cervical (Levels I, II III, IV, or V) or retropharyngeal

M – Distant Metastasis

M0 No distant metastasis
M1 Distant metastasis

pTNM Pathological Classification

The pT and pN categories correspond to the T and N categories. For pM see page 8.

pN0 Histological examination of a selective neck dissection specimen will ordinarily include 6 or more lymph nodes. If the lymph nodes are negative, but the number ordinarily examined is not met, classify as pN0.

Histopathological Types

The four major histopathological types are:
- Papillary carcinoma (including those with follicular foci)
- Follicular carcinoma (including so-called Hürthle cell carcinoma)
- Medullary carcinoma
- Anaplastic

Stage

Separate stage groupings are recommended for papillary and follicular (differentiated), medullary, and anaplastic (undifferentiated) carcinomas:

Papillary and Follicular* under 55 years

Stage I	Any T	Any N	M0
Stage II	Any T	Any N	M1

Papillary or Follicular 55 years and older

Stage I	T1a,T1b,T2	N0	M0
Stage II	T3	N0	M0
	T1,T2,T3	N1	M0
Stage III	T4a	Any N	M0
Stage IVA	T4b	Any N	M0
Stage IVB	Any T	Any N	M1

Medullary

Stage I	T1a,T1b	N0	M0
Stage II	T2,T3	N0	M0
Stage III	T1,T2,T3	N1a	M0
Stage IVA	T1,T2,T3	N1b	M0
	T4a	Any N	M0
Stage IVB	T4b	Any N	M0
Stage IVC	Any T	Any N	M1

Anaplastic

Stage IVA	T1,T2,T3a	N0	M0
Stage IVB	T1,T2,T3a	N1	M0
Stage IVB	T3b,T4a,T4b	N0,N1	M0
Stage IVC	Any T	Any N	M1

Note
* Including papillary, follicular, poorly differentiated, and Hurthle cell carcinomas.

Head & Neck

Prognostic Factor Grid – Papillary and Follicular Thyroid Carcinoma

Prognostic factors for survival in differentiated thyroid carcinoma of follicular cell derivation

Prognostic factors	Tumour related	Host related	Environment related
Essential	Extrathyroid extension (T category) M category Post-treatment thyroglobulin	Age	Residual disease: R0, 1 or 2
Additional	N category Site of metastases *BRAFV600E* mutation	Gender	Extent of resection Iodine ablation Endemic goitre
New and promising	Molecular profile		

Source: UICC Manual of Clinical Oncology, Ninth Edition. Edited by Brian O'Sullivan, James D. Brierley, Anil K. D'Cruz, Martin F. Fey, Raphael Pollock, Jan B. Vermorken and Shao Hui Huang. © 2015 UICC. Published 2015 by John Wiley & Sons, Ltd.

Prognostic Factor Grid – Medullary Cancer

Prognostic factors	Tumour related	Host related	Environment related
Essential	Pre- and postoperative calcitonin and CEA	Age	Extent of resection
Additional	MEN Germline mutation Calcitonin doubling time		
New and promising	Molecular profile		

Digestive System Tumours

Introductory Notes

The following sites and types are included:
- Oesophagus and Oesophagogastric Junction
- Stomach
- Small Intestine
- Appendix
- Colon and Rectum
- Anal Canal and Perianal Skin
- Liver cell carcinoma
- Intrahepatic cholangiocarcinoma
- Gallbladder
- Perihilar Bile Duct
- Distal Extrahepatic Bile Duct
- Ampulla of Vater
- Pancreas
- Neuroendocrine Tumours

Each site is described under the following headings:
- Rules for classification with the procedures for assessing T, N, and M categories; additional methods may be used when they enhance the accuracy of appraisal before treatment
- Anatomical sites and subsites where appropriate
- Definition of the regional lymph nodes
- TNM clinical classification
- pTNM pathological classification
- G Histopathological grading where appropriate
- Stage
- Prognostic factors grid

Digestive System

TNM Classification of Malignant Tumours, Eighth Edition. Edited by James D. Brierley,
Mary K. Gospodarowicz and Christian Wittekind.
© 2017 UICC. Published 2017 by John Wiley & Sons, Ltd.

Regional Lymph Nodes

The number of lymph nodes ordinarily included in a lymphadenectomy specimen is noted at each site.

Oesophagus (ICD-O-3 C15) Including Oesophagogastric Junction (C16.0)

Rules for Classification

The classification applies only to carcinomas and includes adenocarcinomas of the oesophagogastric/gastroesophageal junction. There should be histological confirmation of the disease and division of cases by topographic localization and histological type. A tumour the epicentre of which is within 2 cm of the **oesophagogastric junction** and also extends into the oesophagus is classified and staged using the oesophageal scheme. Cancers involving the oesophagogastric junction (OGJ) whose epicentre is within the proximal 2 cm of the cardia (Siewert types I/II) are to be staged as oesophageal cancers.

The following are the procedures for assessing T, N, and M categories.

T *categories*	Physical examination, imaging, endoscopy (including bronchoscopy), and/or surgical exploration
N *categories*	Physical examination, imaging, and/or surgical exploration
M *categories*	Physical examination, imaging, and/or surgical exploration

Anatomical Subsites

1. Cervical oesophagus (C15.0): this commences at the lower border of the cricoid cartilage and ends at the thoracic inlet (suprasternal notch), approximately 18 cm from the upper incisor teeth.
2. Intrathoracic oesophagus
   a) The upper thoracic portion (C15.3) extending from the thoracic inlet to the level of the tracheal bifurcation, approximately 24 cm from the upper incisor teeth
   b) The mid-thoracic portion (C15.4) is the proximal half of the oesophagus between the tracheal bifurcation and the oesophagogastric junction. The lower level is approximately 32 cm from the upper incisor teeth
   c) The lower thoracic portion (C15.5), approximately 8 cm in length (includes abdominal oesophagus), is the distal half of the oesophagus between the tracheal bifurcation and the oesophagogastric junction. The lower level is approximately 40 cm from the upper incisor teeth

Digestive System

3. Oesophagogastric junction (C16.0). Cancers involving the oesophago-gastric junction (OGJ) whose epicentre is within the proximal 2 cm of the cardia (Siewert types I/II) are to be staged as oesophageal cancers. Cancers whose epicentre is more than 2 cm distal from the OGJ will be staged using the Stomach Cancer TNM and Stage even if the OGJ is involved.

Regional Lymph Nodes

The regional lymph nodes, irrespective of the site of the primary tumour, are those in the oesophageal drainage area including coeliac axis nodes and paraesophageal nodes in the neck but not the supraclavicular nodes.

TNM Clinical Classification

T – Primary Tumour

TX   Primary tumour cannot be assessed
T0   No evidence of primary tumour
Tis   Carcinoma in situ/high-grade dysplasia

T1   Tumour invades lamina propria, muscularis mucosae, or submucosa
    T1a   Tumour invades lamina propria or muscularis mucosae
    T1b   Tumour invades submucosa
T2   Tumour invades muscularis propria
T3   Tumour invades adventitia
T4   Tumour invades adjacent structures
    T4a   Tumour invades pleura, pericardium, azygos vein, diaphragm, or peritoneum
    T4b   Tumour invades other adjacent structures such as aorta, vertebral body, or trachea

N – Regional Lymph Nodes

NX   Regional lymph nodes cannot be assessed
N0   No regional lymph node metastasis
N1   Metastasis in 1 to 2 regional lymph nodes
N2   Metastasis in 3 to 6 regional lymph nodes
N3   Metastasis in 7 or more regional lymph nodes

M – Distant Metastasis

M0   No distant metastasis
M1   Distant metastasis

pTNM Pathological Classification

The pT and pN categories correspond to the T and N categories. For pM see page 8.

pN0 Histological examination of a regional lymphadenectomy specimen will ordinarily include 7 or more lymph nodes. If the lymph nodes are negative, but the number ordinarily examined is not met, classify as pN0.

Stage and Prognostic Group – Carcinomas of the Oesophagus and Oesophagogastric Junction*

Squamous Cell Carcinoma
Clinical Stage

Stage 0	Tis	N0	M0
Stage I	T1	N0, N1	M0
Stage II	T2	N0, N1	M0
	T3	N0	M0
Stage III	T1, T2	N2	M0
	T3	N1, N2	M0
Stage IVA	T4a, T4b	N0, N1, N2	M0
Stage IVA	Any T	N3	M0
Stage IVB	Any T	Any N	M1

Pathological Stage

Stage 0	Tis	N0	M0
Stage IA	T1a	N0	M0
Stage IB	T1b	N0	M0
Stage IIA	T2	N0	M0
Stage IIB	T1	N1	M0
	T3	N0	M0
Stage IIIA	T1	N2	M0
	T2	N1	M0
Stage IIIB	T2	N2	M0
	T3	N1, N2	M0
	T4a	N0, N1	M0
Stage IVA	T4a	N2	M0
	T4b	Any N	M0
	Any T	N3	M0
Stage IV	Any T	Any N	M1

Pathological Prognostic Group

Group	T	N	M	Grade	Location
Group 0	Tis	N0	M0	N/A	Any
Group IA	T1a	N0	M0	1, X	Any
Group IB	T1a	N0	M0	2–3	Any
	T1b	N0	M0	Any	Any
	T2	N0	M0	1	Any
Group IIA	T2	N0	M0	2–3, X	Any
	T3	N0	M0	Any	Lower,
	T3	N0	M0	1	Upper, middle
Group IIB	T3	N0	M0	2–3	Upper, middle
	T3	N0	M0	Any	X
	T3	N0	M0	X	Any
	T1	N1	M0	Any	Any
Group IIIA	T1	N2	M0	Any	Any
	T2	N1	M0	Any	Any
Group IIIB	T2	N2	M0	Any	Any
	T3	N1,N2	M0	Any	Any
	T4a	N0,N1	M0	Any	Any
Group IVA	T4a	N2	M0	Any	Any
	T4b	Any N	M0	Any	Any
	Any T	N3	M0	Any	Any
Group IVB	Any T	Any N	M1	Any	Any

Adenocarcinoma
Clinical Stage

	T	N	M
Stage 0	Tis	N0	M0
Stage I	T1	N0	M0
Stage IIA	T1	N1	M0
Stage IIB	T2	N0	M0
Stage III	T2	N1	M0
	T3,T4a	N0, N1	M0
Stage IVA	T1–T4a	N2	M0
	T4b	N0, N1, N2	M0
	Any T	N3	M0
Stage IVB	Any T	Any N	M1

Pathological Stage

Stage 0	Tis	N0	M0
Stage IA	T1a	N0	M0
Stage IB	T1b	N0	M0
Stage IIA	T2	N0	M0
Stage IIB	T1	N1	M0
	T3	N0	M0
Stage IIIA	T1	N2	M0
	T2	N1	M0
Stage IIIB	T2	N2	M0
	T3	N1, N2	M0
	T4a	N0, N1	M0
Stage IVA	T4a	N2	M0
	T4b	Any N	M0
	Any T	N3	M0
Stage IVB	Any T	Any N	M1

Pathological Prognostic Group

	T	N	M	Grade
Group 0	Tis	N0	M0	N/A
Group IA	T1a	N0	M0	1, X
Group IB	T1a	N0	M0	2,
	T1b	N0	M0	1, 2
Group IC	T1a, T1b	N0	M0	3
	T2	N0	M0	1, 2
Group IIA	T2	N0	M0	3, X
Group IIB	T1	N1	M0	Any
	T3	N0	M0	Any
Group IIIA	T1	N2	M0	Any
	T2	N1	M0	Any
	T3,	N0	M0	Any
Group IIIB	T2	N2	M0	Any
	T3	N1,N2	M0	Any
	T4a	N0,N1	M0	Any

	T	N	M	Grade
Group IVA	T4a	N2	M0	Any
	T4b	Any N	M0	Any
	Any T	N3	M0	Any
Group IVB	Any T	Any N	M1	Any

Note

* The AJCC publishes prognostic groups for adenocarcinoma and squamous cell carcinoma after neoadjuvant therapy (categories with the prefix "y").

Prognostic Factors Grid – Oesophagus

Prognostic factors for survival in oesophageal cancer

Prognostic factors	Tumour related	Host related	Treatment related
Essential	Depth of invasion Lymph node involvement Presence of lymphovascular invasion (LVI)	Performance status Age Nutritional status	Quality of surgery Multimodality approach
Additional	Tumour grading Tumour location	Economic status	Nutritional support
New and promising	CEA, VEGF-C, HER2		

Source: UICC Manual of Clinical Oncology, Ninth Edition. Edited by Brian O'Sullivan, James D. Brierley, Anil K. D'Cruz, Martin F. Fey, Raphael Pollock, Jan B. Vermorken and Shao Hui Huang. © 2015 UICC. Published 2015 by John Wiley & Sons, Ltd.

Stomach
(ICD-O-3 C16)

Rules for Classification

The classification applies only to carcinomas. There should be histological confirmation of the disease. Cancers involving the oesophagogastric junction (OGJ) whose epicentre is within the proximal 2 cm of the cardia (Siewert types I/II) are to be staged as oesophageal cancers. Cancers whose epicentre is more than 2 cm distal from the OGJ will be staged using the Stomach Cancer TNM and Stage even if the OGJ is involved.

Changes in this edition from the seventh edition are based upon recommendations from the International Gastric Cancer Association Staging Project.[1]

The following are the procedures for assessing T, N, and M categories.

T categories   Physical examination, imaging, endoscopy, and/or surgical exploration

N categories   Physical examination, imaging, and/or surgical exploration

M categories   Physical examination, imaging, and/or surgical exploration

Anatomical Subsites

1. Cardia (16.0)
2. Fundus (C16.1)
3. Corpus (C16.2)
4. Antrum (C16.3) and pylorus (C16.4)

Regional Lymph Nodes

The regional lymph nodes of the stomach are the perigastric nodes along the lesser and greater curvatures, the nodes along the left gastric, common hepatic, splenic, and coeliac arteries, and the hepatoduodenal nodes.

Involvement of other intra-abdominal lymph nodes such as retropancreatic, mesenteric, and para-aortic is classified as distant metastasis.

TNM Clinical Classification

T – Primary Tumour

TX   Primary tumour cannot be assessed
T0   No evidence of primary tumour

Digestive System

Tis   Carcinoma in situ: intraepithelial tumour without invasion of the lamina propria, high-grade dysplasia

T1   Tumour invades lamina propria, muscularis mucosae, or submucosa
    T1a   Tumour invades lamina propria or muscularis mucosae
    T1b   Tumour invades submucosa
T2   Tumour invades muscularis propria
T3   Tumour invades subserosa
T4   Tumour perforates serosa (visceral peritoneum) or invades adjacent structures[a, b, c]
    T4a   Tumour perforates serosa
    T4b   Tumour invades adjacent structures[a, b]

Notes
[a] The adjacent structures of the stomach are the spleen, transverse colon, liver, diaphragm, pancreas, abdominal wall, adrenal gland, kidney, small intestine, and retroperitoneum.
[b] Intramural extension to the duodenum or oesophagus is classified by the depth of greatest invasion in any of these sites including stomach.
[c] Tumour that extends into gastrocolic or gastrohepatic ligaments or into greater or lesser omentum, without perforation of visceral peritoneum, is T3.

N – Regional Lymph Nodes

NX   Regional lymph nodes cannot be assessed
N0   No regional lymph node metastasis
N1   Metastasis in 1 to 2 regional lymph nodes
N2   Metastasis in 3 to 6 regional lymph nodes
N3   Metastasis in 7 or more regional lymph nodes
    N3a   Metastasis in 7 to 15 regional lymph nodes
    N3b   Metastasis in 16 or more regional lymph nodes

M – Distant Metastasis

M0   No distant metastasis
M1   Distant metastasis

Note
Distant metastasis includes peritoneal seeding, positive peritoneal cytology, and omental tumour not part of continuous extension.

ptNM Pathological Classification

he pT and pN categories correspond to the T and N categories. For pM see page 8.

pN0   Histological examination of a regional lymphadenectomy specimen will ordinarily include 16 or more lymph nodes. If the lymph nodes are negative, but the number ordinarily examined is not met, classify as pN0.

Clinical Stage

Stage I	T1, T2	N0	M0
Stage IIA	T1, T2	N1, N2, N3	M0
Stage IIB	T3, T4a	N0	M0
Stage III	T3, T4a	N1, N2, N3	M0
Stage IVA	T4b	Any N	M0
Stage IVB	Any T	Any N	M1

Pathological Stage*

Stage 0	Tis	N0	M0
Stage IA	T1	N0	M0
Stage IB	T1	N1	M0
	T2	N0	M0
Stage IIA	T1	N2	M0
	T2	N1	M0
	T3	N0	M0
Stage IIB	T1	N3a	M0
	T2	N2	M0
	T3	N1	M0
	T4a	N0	M0
Stage IIIA	T2	N3a	M0
	T3	N2	M0
	T4a	N1, N2	M0
	T4b	N0	M0
Stage IIIB	T1, T2	N3b	M0
	T3, T4a	N3a	M0
	T4b	N1, N2	M0
Stage IIIC	T3, T4a	N3b	M0
	T4b	N3a, N3b	M0
Stage IV	Any T	Any N	M1

Note

* The AJCC publishes prognostic groups for after neoadjuvant therapy (categories with the prefix "y").

Prognostic Factor Grid – Stomach

Prognostic factors for survival in gastric adenocarcinoma

Prognostic factors	Tumour related	Host related	Environment related
Essential	T category N category M category HER2 status		Residual disease: R0, R1 or R2
Additional	Tumour site: cardia or distal stomach Histological type Vessel infiltration	Age	Extent of resection
New and promising	Molecular profile	Race: Asian or non-Asian	

Source: UICC Manual of Clinical Oncology, Ninth Edition. Edited by Brian O'Sullivan, James D. Brierley, Anil K. D'Cruz, Martin F. Fey, Raphael Pollock, Jan B. Vermorken and Shao Hui Huang. © 2015 UICC. Published 2015 by John Wiley & Sons, Ltd.

Reference

1 Sano T, Coit D, Kim HH, et al. for the IGCA Staging Project. Proposal of a new stage grouping of gastric cancer for TNM classification: International Gastric Cancer Association Staging Project. *Gastric Cancer* 2016; in press.

Small Intestine
(ICD-O-3 C17)

Rules for Classification

The classification applies only to carcinomas. There should be histological confirmation of the disease.

The following are the procedures for assessing T, N, and M categories.

T categories   Physical examination, imaging, endoscopy, and/or surgical exploration

N categories   Physical examination, imaging, and/or surgical exploration

M categories   Physical examination, imaging, and/or surgical exploration

Anatomical Subsites

1. Duodenum (C17.0)
2. Jejunum (C17.1)
3. Ileum (C17.2) (excludes ileocecal valve C18.0)

Note

This classification does not apply to carcinomas of the ampulla of Vater (see page 91).

Regional Lymph Nodes

The regional lymph nodes for the duodenum are the pancreaticoduodenal, pyloric, hepatic (pericholedochal, cystic, hilar), and superior mesenteric nodes.

The regional lymph nodes for the ileum and jejunum are the mesenteric nodes, including the superior mesenteric nodes, and, for the terminal ileum only, the ileocolic nodes including the posterior caecal nodes.

TNM Clinical Classification

T – Primary Tumour

TX   Primary tumour cannot be assessed
T0   No evidence of primary tumour
Tis   Carcinoma in situ

Digestive System

T1 Tumour invades lamina propria, muscularis mucosae or submucosa

  T1a Tumour invades lamina propria or muscularis mucosae

  T1b Tumour invades submucosa

T2 Tumour invades muscularis propria

T3 Tumour invades subserosa or non-peritonealized perimuscular tissue (mesentery or retroperitoneum*) without perforation of the serosa

T4 Tumour perforates visceral peritoneum or directly invades other organs or structures (includes other loops of small intestine, mesentery, or retroperitoneum and abdominal wall by way of serosa; for duodenum only, invasion of pancreas)

Note

* The non-peritonealized perimuscular tissue is, for jejunum and ileum, part of the mesentery and, for duodenum in areas where serosa is lacking, part of the retroperitoneum.

N – Regional Lymph Nodes

NX Regional lymph nodes cannot be assessed

N0 No regional lymph node metastasis

N1 Metastasis in 1 to 2 regional lymph nodes

N2 Metastasis in 3 or more regional lymph nodes

M – Distant Metastasis

M0 No distant metastasis

M1 Distant metastasis

pTNM Pathological Classification

The pT and pN categories correspond to the T and N categories. For pM see page 8.

pN0 Histological examination of a regional lymphadenectomy specimen will ordinarily include 6 or more lymph nodes. If the lymph nodes are negative, but the number ordinarily examined is not met, classify as pN0.

Stage

Stage 0	Tis	N0	M0
Stage I	T1, T2	N0	M0
Stage IIA	T3	N0	M0
Stage IIB	T4	N0	M0
Stage IIIA	Any T	N1	M0
Stage IIIB	Any T	N2	M0
Stage IV	Any T	Any N	M1

Appendix
(ICD-O-3 C18.1)

Rules for Classification

The classification applies to adenocarcinomas of the appendix. Neuroendocrine carcinomas are classified separately (page 97). There should be histological confirmation of the disease and separation of carcinomas into mucinous and non-mucinous adenocarcinomas.

Goblet cell carcinoids are classified according to the carcinoma scheme.

Grading is of particular importance for mucinous tumours.

The following are the procedures for assessing T, N, and M categories.

T *categories*	Physical examination, imaging, and/or surgical exploration
N *categories*	Physical examination, imaging, and/or surgical exploration
M *categories*	Physical examination, imaging, and/or surgical exploration

Anatomical Site

Appendix (C18.1)

Regional Lymph Nodes

The ileocolic are the regional lymph nodes.

TNM Clinical Classification

T – Primary Tumour

TX	Primary tumour cannot be assessed
T0	No evidence of primary tumour
Tis	Carcinoma in situ: intraepithelial or invasion of lamina propria[a]
Tis (LAMN)	Low-grade appendiceal mucinous neoplasm confined to the appendix (defined as involvement by acellular mucin or mucinous epithelium that may extend into muscularis propria)
T1	Tumour invades submucosa
T2	Tumour invades muscularis propria
T3	Tumour invades subserosa or mesoappendix
T4	Tumour perforates visceral peritoneum, including mucinous peritoneal tumour or acellular mucin on the serosa of the

appendix or mesoappendix and/or directly invades other organs or structures[b,c,d]

T4a   Tumour perforates visceral peritoneum, including mucinous peritoneal tumour or acellular mucin on the serosa of the appendix or mesoappendix

T4b   Tumour directly invades other organs or structures

Notes

[a] Tis includes cancer cells confined within the glandular basement membrane (intraepithelial) or lamina propria (intramucosal) with no extension through muscularis mucosae into submucosa.

[b] Direct invasion in T4 includes invasion of other intestinal segments by way of the serosa, e.g., invasion of ileum.

[c] Tumour that is adherent to other organs or structures, macroscopically, is classified cT4b. However, if no tumour is present in the adhesion, microscopically, the classification should be pT1, 2, or 3.

[d] LAMN with involvement of the subserosa or the serosal surface (visceral peritoneum) should be classified as T3 or T4a respectively.

N – Regional Lymph Nodes

NX   Regional lymph nodes cannot be assessed
N0   No regional lymph node metastasis
N1   Metastasis in 1 to 3 regional lymph nodes
 N1a   Metastases in 1 regional lymph node
 N1b   Metastases in 2–3 regional lymph nodes
 N1c   Tumour deposit(s), i.e. satellites,* in the subserosa, or in non-peritonealized pericolic or perirectal soft tissue without regional lymph node metastasis
N2   Metastasis in 4 or more regional lymph nodes

Note

* Tumour deposits (satellites) are discrete macroscopic or microscopic nodules of cancer in the pericolorectal adipose tissue's lymph drainage area of a primary carcinoma that are discontinuous from the primary and without histological evidence of residual lymph node or identifiable vascular or neural structures. If a vessel wall is identifiable on H&E, elastic or other stains, it should be classified as venous invasion (V1/2) or lymphatic invasion (L1). Similarly, if neural structures are identifiable, the lesion should be classified as perineural invasion (Pn1).

M – Distant Metastasis

M0   No distant metastasis
M1   Distant metastasis
    M1a   Intraperitoneal acellular mucin only
    M1b   Intraperitoneal metastasis only, including mucinous epithelium
    M1c   Non-peritoneal metastasis

pTNM Pathological Classification

The pT and pN categories correspond to the T and N categories. For pM see page 8.

pN0   Histological examination of a regional lymphadenectomy specimen will ordinarily include 12 or more lymph nodes. If the lymph nodes are negative, but the number ordinarily examined is not met, classify as pN0.

Stage

Stage 0	Tis	N0	M0	
Stage 0	Tis(LAMN)	N0	M0	
Stage I	T1, T2	N0	M0	
Stage IIA	T3	N0	M0	
IIB	T4a	N0	M0	
IIC	T4b	N0	M0	
Stage IIIA	T1, T2	N1	M0	
IIIB	T3, T4	N1	M0	
IIIC	Any T	N2	M0	
Stage IVA	Any T	N0	M1a	
	Any T	N0	M1b	G1
IVB	Any T	Any N	M1b	G2, G3, GX
Stage IVC	Any T	Any N	M1c	Any G

Colon and Rectum
(ICD-O-3 C18-20)

Rules for Classification

The classification applies only to carcinomas. There should be histological confirmation of the disease.

The following are the procedures for assessing the T, N, and M categories.

T *categories*   Physical examination, imaging, endoscopy, and/or surgical exploration

N *categories*   Physical examination, imaging, and/or surgical exploration

M *categories*   Physical examination, imaging, and/or surgical exploration

Anatomical Sites and Subsites

Colon (C18)
1. Caecum (C18.0)
2. Ascending colon (C18.2)
3. Hepatic flexure (C18.3)
4. Transverse colon (C18.4)
5. Splenic flexure (C18.5)
6. Descending colon (C18.6)
7. Sigmoid colon (C18.7)

Rectosigmoid junction (C19)
Rectum (C20)

Regional Lymph Nodes

For each anatomical site or subsite the following are regional lymph nodes:

Caecum	ileocolic, right colic
Ascending colon	ileocolic, right colic, middle colic
Hepatic flexure	right colic, middle colic
Transverse colon	right colic, middle colic, left colic, inferior mesenteric
Splenic flexure	middle colic, left colic, inferior mesenteric
Descending colon	left colic, inferior mesenteric
Sigmoid colon	sigmoid, left colic, superior rectal (haemorrhoidal), inferior mesenteric and rectosigmoid

Digestive System

Rectum   superior, middle, and inferior rectal (haemorrhoidal), inferior mesenteric, internal iliac, mesorectal (paraproctal), lateral sacral, presacral, sacral promontory (Gerota)

Metastasis in nodes other than those listed here is classified as distant metastasis.

TNM Clinical Classification

T – Primary Tumour

TX   Primary tumour cannot be assessed
T0   No evidence of primary tumour
■ Tis   Carcinoma in situ: invasion of lamina propria[a]

T1   Tumour invades submucosa
T2   Tumour invades muscularis propria
T3   Tumour invades subserosa or into non-peritonealized pericolic or perirectal tissues
T4   Tumour directly invades other organs or structures[b,c,d] and/or perforates visceral peritoneum
    T4a   Tumour perforates visceral peritoneum
    T4b   Tumour directly invades other organs or structures

Notes

[a] Tis includes cancer cells confined within the mucosal lamina propria (intramucosal) with no extension through the muscularis mucosae into the submucosa.

[b] Invades through to visceral peritoneum to involve the surface.

[c] Direct invasion in T4b includes invasion of other organs or segments of the colorectum by way of the serosa, as confirmed on microscopic examination, or for tumours in a retroperitoneal or subperitoneal location, direct invasion of other organs or structures by virtue of extension beyond the muscularis propria.

[d] Tumour that is adherent to other organs or structures, macroscopically, is classified cT4b. However, if no tumour is present in the adhesion, microscopically, the classification should be pT1-3, depending on the anatomical depth of wall invasion.

N – Regional Lymph Nodes

NX   Regional lymph nodes cannot be assessed
N0   No regional lymph node metastasis

N1   Metastasis in 1 to 3 regional lymph nodes
    N1a   Metastasis in 1 regional lymph node
    N1b   Metastasis in 2 to 3 regional lymph nodes
    N1c   Tumour deposit(s), i.e. satellites,* in the subserosa, or in non-peritonealized pericolic or perirectal soft tissue *without* regional lymph node metastasis
N2   Metastasis in 4 or more regional lymph nodes
    N2a   Metastasis in 4–6 regional lymph nodes
    N2b   Metastasis in 7 or more regional lymph nodes

Note

* Tumour deposits (satellites) are discrete macroscopic or microscopic nodules of cancer in the pericolorectal adipose tissue's lymph drainage area of a primary carcinoma that are discontinuous from the primary and without histological evidence of residual lymph node or identifiable vascular or neural structures. If a vessel wall is identifiable on H&E, elastic or other stains, it should be classified as venous invasion (V1/2) or lymphatic invasion (L1). Similarly, if neural structures are identifiable, the lesion should be classified as perineural invasion (Pn1). The presence of tumour deposits does not change the primary tumour T category, but changes the node status (N) to pN1c if all regional lymph nodes are negative on pathological examination.

M – Distant Metastasis

M0   No distant metastasis
M1   Distant metastasis
    M1a   Metastasis confined to one organ (liver, lung, ovary, non-regional lymph node(s)) without peritoneal metastases
    M1b   Metastasis in more than one organ
    M1c   Metastasis to the peritoneum with or without other organ involvement

TNM Pathological Classification

The pT and pN categories correspond to the T and N categories. For pM see page 8.
pN0   Histological examination of a regional lymphadenectomy specimen will ordinarily include 12 or more lymph nodes. If the lymph nodes are negative, but the number ordinarily examined is not met, classify as pN0.

Stage

Stage 0	Tis	N0	M0
Stage I	T1, T2	N0	M0
Stage II	T3, T4	N0	M0
Stage IIA	T3	N0	M0
Stage IIB	T4a	N0	M0
Stage IIC	T4b	N0	M0
Stage III	Any T	N1, N2	M0
Stage IIIA	T1, T2	N1	M0
	T1	N2a	M0
Stage IIIB	T1, T2	N2b	M0
	T2, T3	N2a	M0
	T3, T4a	N1	M0
Stage IIIC	T3, T4a	N2b	M0
	T4a	N2a	M0
	T4b	N1, N2	M0
Stage IV	Any T	Any N	M1
Stage IVA	Any T	Any N	M1a
Stage IVB	Any T	Any N	M1b
Stage IVC	Any T	Any N	M1c

Prognostic Factors Grid – Colon and Rectum

Prognostic factors for survival in differentiated colorectal cancer

Prognostic factors	Tumour related	Host related	Environment related
Essential	T category N category M category Circumferential margin (rectal cancer)	Age	Screening programme
Additional	Vascular/lymphatic invasion Perineural invasion Grade Tumour budding Perforation *KRAS* MSI *BRAF*	Race	Socioeconomic status Centre volume and experience
New and promising	Molecular profile		

Source: UICC Manual of Clinical Oncology, Ninth Edition. Edited by Brian O'Sullivan, James D. Brierley, Anil K. D'Cruz, Martin F. Fey, Raphael Pollock, Jan B. Vermorken and Shao Hui Huang. © 2015 UICC. Published 2015 by John Wiley & Sons, Ltd.

Anal Canal and Perianal Skin
(ICD-O-3 C21, ICD-O-3 C44.5)

The anal canal extends from rectum to perianal skin (to the junction with hair-bearing skin). It is lined by the mucous membrane overlying the internal sphincter, including the transitional epithelium and dentate line. Tumours of anal margin and perianal skin defined as within 5 cm of the anal margin (ICD-O C44.5) are now classified with carcinomas of the anal canal.

Rules for Classification

The classification applies only to carcinomas. There should be histological confirmation of the disease and division of cases by histological type.

The following are the procedures for assessing T, N, and M categories.

T *categories*	Physical examination, imaging, endoscopy, and/or surgical exploration
N *categories*	Physical examination, imaging, and/or surgical exploration
M *categories*	Physical examination, imaging, and/or surgical exploration

Regional Lymph Nodes

The regional lymph nodes are the perirectal, the internal iliac, external iliac, and the inguinal lymph nodes.

TNM Clinical Classification

T – Primary Tumour

TX   Primary tumour cannot be assessed
T0   No evidence of primary tumour
Tis   Carcinoma in *situ*, Bowen disease, high-grade squamous intraepithelial lesion (HSIL), anal intraepithelial neoplasia II–III (AIN II–III)

T1   Tumour 2 cm or less in greatest dimension
T2   Tumour more than 2 cm but not more than 5 cm in greatest dimension
T3   Tumour more than 5 cm in greatest dimension
T4   Tumour of any size invades adjacent organ(s), e.g., vagina, urethra, bladder*

Digestive System

Note

* Direct invasion of the rectal wall, perianal skin, subcutaneous tissue, or the sphincter muscle(s) *alone* is not classified as T4.

N – Regional Lymph Nodes

NX   Regional lymph nodes cannot be assessed

N0   No regional lymph node metastasis

N1   Metastasis in regional lymph node(s)

     N1a   Metastases in inguinal, mesorectal, and/or internal iliac nodes

     N1b   Metastases in external iliac nodes

     N1c   Metastases in external iliac and in inguinal, mesorectal and/or internal iliac nodes

M – Distant Metastasis

M0   No distant metastasis

M1   Distant metastasis

pTNM Pathological Classification

The pT and pN categories correspond to the T and N categories. For pM see page 8.

pN0   Histological examination of a regional perirectal/pelvic lymphadenectomy specimen will ordinarily include 12 or more lymph nodes; histological examination of an inguinal lymphadenectomy specimen will ordinarily include 6 or more lymph nodes. If the lymph nodes are negative, but the number ordinarily examined is not met, classify as pN0.

Stage

Stage 0	Tis	N0	M0
Stage I	T1	N0	M0
Stage IIA	T2	N0	M0
Stage IIB	T3	N0	M0
Stage IIIA	T1, T2,	N1	M0
Stage IIIB	T4	N0	M0
Stage IIIC	T3, T4	N1	M0
Stage IV	Any T	Any N	M1

Prognostic Factors Grid – Anal Canal

Prognostic factors for outcome in anal cancer

Prognostic factors	Tumour related	Host related	Environment related
Essential	T, N and M category	Age Male gender	Cigarette smoking Social deprivation
Additional	Skin ulceration Sphincter involvement Primary tumour size >5 cm	Immune suppression Long-term corticosteroids HIV	
New and promising	Squamous cell carcinoma antigen (SCCAg)	Concomitant herpes simplex virus (HSV) Haemoglobin level	

Source: UICC Manual of Clinical Oncology, Ninth Edition. Edited by Brian O'Sullivan, James D. Brierley, Anil K. D'Cruz, Martin F. Fey, Raphael Pollock, Jan B. Vermorken and Shao Hui Huang. © 2015 UICC. Published 2015 by John Wiley & Sons, Ltd.

Digestive System

Liver
(ICD-O-3 C 22.0)

Rules for Classification

The classification applies to hepatocellular carcinoma.

Cholangio- (intrahepatic bile duct) carcinoma of the liver has a separate classification (see page 83). There should be histological confirmation of the disease.

The following are the procedures for assessing T, N, and M categories.

T *categories*   Physical examination, imaging, and/or surgical exploration
N *categories*   Physical examination, imaging, and/or surgical exploration
M *categories*   Physical examination, imaging, and/or surgical exploration

Note
Although the presence of cirrhosis is an important prognostic factor it does not affect the TNM classification, being an independent prognostic variable.

Regional Lymph Nodes

The regional lymph nodes are the hilar, hepatic (along the proper hepatic artery), periportal (along the portal vein), inferior phrenic, and caval nodes.

TNM Clinical Classification

T – Primary Tumour

TX   Primary tumour cannot be assessed
T0   No evidence of primary tumour

T1a   Solitary tumour 2 cm or less in greatest dimension with or without vascular invasion
T1b   Solitary tumour more than 2 cm in greatest dimension without vascular invasion
T2   Solitary tumour with vascular invasion more than 2 cm dimension or multiple tumours, none more than 5 cm in greatest dimension
T3   Multiple tumours any more than 5 cm in greatest dimension
T4   Tumour(s) involving a major branch of the portal or hepatic vein with direct invasion of adjacent organs (including the diaphragm), other than the gallbladder or with perforation of visceral peritoneum

N – Regional Lymph Nodes

NX   Regional lymph nodes cannot be assessed
N0   No regional lymph node metastasis
N1   Regional lymph node metastasis

M – Distant Metastasis

M0   No distant metastasis
M1   Distant metastasis

pTNM Pathological Classification

The pT and pN categories correspond to the T and N categories. For pM see page 8.

pN0   Histological examination of a regional lymphadenectomy specimen will ordinarily include 3 or more lymph nodes. If the lymph nodes are negative, but the number ordinarily examined is not met, classify as pN0.

Stage – Liver

Stage IA	T1a	N0	M0
Stage IB	T1b	N0	M0
Stage II	T2	N0	M0
Stage IIIA	T3	N0	M0
Stage IIIB	T4	N0	M0
Stage IVA	Any T	N1	M0
Stage IVB	Any T	Any N	M1

Digestive System

Prognostic Factors Grid – Liver

Prognostic factors for liver cancer (HCC)

Prognostic factors	Tumour related	Host related	Environment related
Essential	Major vascular invasion* Microvascular invasion* Size >5 cm Multiple (vs single) Tumour differentiation	Fibrosis of underlying liver* Tumour growth rate Patient performance status at diagnosis Liver function Degree of portal hypertension	Treatment factors: Post-resection residual disease (R0, R1, R2) Post-ablation residual disease Post-embolization residual disease
Additional	AFP level DCP/PIVKA-II level	Hepatitis activity	
New and promising	5-gene score (genetic profile) Cancer stem cell markers Circulating microRNA, DNA, circulating cancer cells	IGF-1 combined with CLIP Regulatory T cells C-reactive protein (CRP), interleukin 10 (IL-10), vascular endothelial growth factor (VEGF), neutrophilto-lymphocyte ratio, MnSOD (magnesium superoxide dismutase)	

* Dominant prognostic factors in resected/transplanted patients.

Source: UICC Manual of Clinical Oncology, Ninth Edition. Edited by Brian O'Sullivan, James D. Brierley, Anil K. D'Cruz, Martin F. Fey, Raphael Pollock, Jan B. Vermorken and Shao Hui Huang. © 2015 UICC. Published 2015 by John Wiley & Sons, Ltd.

Intrahepatic Bile Ducts
(ICD-O-3 C22.1)

Rules for Classification

The staging system applies to intrahepatic cholangiocarcinoma, cholangio-cellular carcinoma, and combined hepatocellular and cholangiocarcinoma (mixed hepatocellular/cholangiocellular carcinoma).

The following are the procedures for assessing T, N, and M categories.

T categories	Physical examination, imaging, and/or surgical exploration
N categories	Physical examination, imaging, and/or surgical exploration
M categories	Physical examination, imaging, and/or surgical exploration

Regional Lymph Nodes

For right-liver intrahepatic cholangiocarcinoma, the regional lymph nodes include the hilar (common bile duct, hepatic artery, portal vein, and cystic duct), periduodenal, and peripancreatic lymph nodes.

For left-liver intrahepatic cholangiocarcinoma, regional lymph nodes include hilar and gastrohepatic lymph nodes.

For intrahepatic cholangiocarcinoma, spread to the coeliac and/or peri-aortic and caval lymph nodes are distant metastases (M1).

TNM Clinical Classification

T – Primary Tumour

TX	Primary tumour cannot be assessed
T0	No evidence of primary tumour
Tis	Carcinoma in situ (intraductal tumour)

T1a	Solitary tumour 5 cm or less in greatest dimension without vascular invasion
T1b	Solitary tumour more than 5 cm in greatest dimension without vascular invasion
T2	Solitary tumour with intrahepatic vascular invasion or multiple tumours, with or without vascular invasion
T3	Tumour perforating the visceral peritoneum
T4	Tumour involving local extrahepatic structures by direct hepatic invasion

N – Regional Lymph Nodes

NX   Regional lymph nodes cannot be assessed
N0   No regional lymph node metastasis
N1   Regional lymph node metastasis

M – Distant Metastasis

M0   No distant metastasis
M1   Distant metastasis

pTNM Pathological Classification

The pT and pN categories correspond to the T and N categories. For pM see page 8.

pN0   Histological examination of a regional lymphadenectomy specimen will ordinarily include 6 or more lymph nodes. If the regional lymph nodes are negative, but the number ordinarily examined is not met, classify as pN0.

Stage – Intrahepatic Bile Ducts

Stage I	T1	N0	M0
Stage IA	T1a	N0	M0
Stage IB	T1b	N0	M0
Stage II	T2	N0	M0
Stage IIIA	T3	N0	M0
Stage IIIB	T4	N0	M0
	Any T	N1	M0
Stage IV	Any T	Any N	M1

Gallbladder
(ICD-O-3 C23.0 and C24.0)

Rules for Classification

The classification applies only to carcinomas of gallbladder (C23.0) and cystic duct (C24.0). There should be histological confirmation of the disease.

The following are the procedures for assessing T, N, and M categories.

T categories	Physical examination, imaging, and/or surgical exploration
N categories	Physical examination, imaging, and/or surgical exploration
M categories	Physical examination, imaging, and/or surgical exploration

Regional Lymph Nodes

Regional lymph nodes are the hepatic hilus nodes (including nodes along the common bile duct, hepatic artery, portal vein, and cystic duct), coeliac, and superior mesenteric artery nodes.

TNM Clinical Classification

T – Primary Tumour

TX	Primary tumour cannot be assessed
T0	No evidence of primary tumour
Tis	Carcinoma in situ

T1   Tumour invades lamina propria or muscular layer

    T1a   Tumour invades lamina propria

    T1b   Tumour invades muscular layer

T2   Tumour invades perimuscular connective tissue; no extension beyond serosa or into liver

    T2a   Tumour invades perimuscular connective tissue on the peritoneal side with no extension to the serosa

    T2b   Tumour invades perimuscular connective tissue on the hepatic side with no extension into the liver

T3   Tumour perforates the serosa (visceral peritoneum) and/or directly invades the liver and/or one other adjacent organ or structure, such as stomach, duodenum, colon, pancreas, omentum, extrahepatic bile ducts

T4   Tumour invades main portal vein or hepatic artery or invades two or more extrahepatic organs or structures

Digestive System

N – Regional Lymph Nodes

NX   Regional lymph nodes cannot be assessed
N0   No regional lymph node metastasis
N1   Metastases to 1–3 regional nodes
N2   Metastasis to 4 or more regional nodes

M – Distant Metastasis

M0   No distant metastasis
M1   Distant metastasis

pTNM Pathological Classification

The pT and pN categories correspond to the T and N categories. For pM see page 8.

pN0   Histological examination of a regional lymphadenectomy specimen will ordinarily include 6 or more lymph nodes. If the regional lymph nodes are negative, but the number ordinarily examined is not met, classify as pN0.

Stage – Gallbladder

Stage 0	Tis	N0	M0
Stage IA	T1a	N0	M0
Stage IB	T1b	N0	M0
Stage IIA	T2a	N0	M0
Stage IIB	T2b	N0	M0
Stage IIIA	T3	N0	M0
Stage IIIB	T1, T2, T3	N1	M0
Stage IVA	T4	N0, N1	M0
Stage IVB	Any T	N2	M0
	Any T	Any N	M1

Perihilar Bile Ducts
(ICD-O-3 C24.0)

Rules for Classification

The classification applies to carcinomas of the extrahepatic bile ducts of perihilar localization (Klatskin tumour). Included are the right, left and the common hepatic ducts.

The following are the procedures for assessing T, N, and M categories.

T *categories*   Physical examination, imaging, and/or surgical exploration
N *categories*   Physical examination, imaging, and/or surgical exploration
M *categories*   Physical examination, imaging, and/or surgical exploration

Anatomical Sites and Subsites

Perihilar cholangiocarcinomas are tumours located in the extrahepatic biliary tree proximal to the origin of the cystic duct.

Regional Lymph Nodes

The regional nodes are the hilar and pericholedochal nodes in the hepatoduodenal ligament.

TNM Clinical Classification

T – Primary Tumour

TX   Primary tumour cannot be assessed
T0   No evidence of primary tumour
Tis   Carcinoma in situ

T1   Tumour confined to the bile duct, with extension up to the muscle layer or fibrous tissue
T2a   Tumour invades beyond the wall of the bile duct to surrounding adipose tissue
T2b   Tumour invades adjacent hepatic parenchyma
T3   Tumour invades unilateral branches of the portal vein or hepatic artery
T4   Tumour invades the main portal vein or its branches bilaterally; or the common hepatic artery; or unilateral second-order biliary radicals with contralateral portal vein or hepatic artery involvement

N – Regional Lymph Nodes

NX   Regional lymph nodes cannot be assessed
N0   No regional lymph node metastasis
N1   Metastases to 1–3 regional lymph nodes
N2   Metastases to 4 or more regional nodes

M – Distant Metastasis

M0   No distant metastasis
M1   Distant metastasis

pTNM Pathological Classification

The pT and pN categories correspond to the T and N categories. For pM see page 8.

pN0   Histological examination of a regional lymphadenectomy specimen will ordinarily include 15 more lymph nodes. If the regional lymph nodes are negative, but the number ordinarily examined is not met, classify as pN0.

Stage – Perihilar Bile Ducts

Stage 0	Tis	N0	M0
Stage I	T1	N0	M0
Stage II	T2a, T2b	N0	M0
Stage IIIA	T3	N0	M0
Stage IIIB	T4	N0	M0
Stage IIIC	Any T	N1	M0
Stage IVA	Any T	N2	M0
Stage IVB	Any T	Any N	M1

Distal Extrahepatic Bile Duct (ICD-O-3 C24.0)

Rules for Classification

The classification applies to carcinomas of the extrahepatic bile ducts distal to the insertion of the cystic duct. Cystic duct carcinoma is included under gallbladder.

The following are the procedures for assessing T, N, and M categories.

T *categories*   Physical examination, imaging, and/or surgical exploration
N *categories*   Physical examination, imaging, and/or surgical exploration
M *categories*   Physical examination, imaging, and/or surgical exploration

Regional Lymph Nodes

The regional lymph nodes are along the common bile duct, hepatic artery, back towards the coeliac trunk, posterior and anterior pancreaticoduodenal nodes, and nodes along the superior mesenteric artery

TNM Clinical Classification

T – Primary Tumour

TX   Primary tumour cannot be assessed
T0   No evidence of primary tumour
Tis   Carcinoma *in situ*

T1   Tumour invades bile duct wall to a depth less than 5 mm
T2   Tumour invades bile duct wall to a depth of 5 mm up to 12 mm
T3   Tumour invades bile duct wall to a depth of more than 12 mm
T4   Tumour involves the coeliac axis, the superior mesenteric artery and/or the common hepatic artery

N – Regional Lymph Nodes

NX   Regional lymph nodes cannot be assessed
N1   Metastases to 1–3 regional nodes
N2   Metastasis to 4 or more regional nodes

Digestive System

M – Distant Metastasis

M0   No distant metastasis
M1   Distant metastasis

pTNM Pathological Classification

The pT and pN categories correspond to the T and N categories. For pM see page 8.

pN0   Histological examination of a regional lymphadenectomy specimen will ordinarily include 12 or more lymph nodes. If the regional lymph nodes are negative, but the number ordinarily examined is not met, classify as pN0.

Stage – Distal Extrahepatic Bile Duct

Stage 0	Tis	N0	M0
Stage I	T1	N0	M0
Stage IIA	T1	N1	M0
	T2	N0	M0
Stage IIB	T2	N1	M0
	T3	N0, N1	M0
Stage IIIA	T1, T2, T3	N2	M0
Stage IIIB	T4	Any N	M0
Stage IV	Any T	Any N	M1

Prognostic Factor Grid – Biliary Tract and Gallbladder Cancers

Prognostic risk factors in biliary tract carcinoma

Prognostic factors	Tumour related	Host related	Environment related
Essential	Resectable	ECOG status	Residual disease (R0, R1, R2)
Additional	Lymph node metastases		
New and promising	FGFR2 mutations		

Source: UICC Manual of Clinical Oncology, Ninth Edition. Edited by Brian O'Sullivan, James D. Brierley, Anil K. D'Cruz, Martin F. Fey, Raphael Pollock, Jan B. Vermorken and Shao Hui Huang. © 2015 UICC. Published 2015 by John Wiley & Sons, Ltd.

Ampulla of Vater
(ICD-O C24.1)

Rules for Classification

The classification applies only to carcinomas. There should be histological confirmation of the disease.

The following are the procedures for assessing T, N, and M categories.

T *categories*	Physical examination, imaging, and/or surgical exploration
N *categories*	Physical examination, imaging, and/or surgical exploration
M *categories*	Physical examination, imaging, and/or surgical exploration

Regional Lymph Nodes

The regional lymph nodes are the same as for the head of the pancreas and are the lymph nodes along the common bile duct, common hepatic artery, portal vein, pyloric, infrapyloric, subpyloric, proximal mesenteric, coeliac, posterior and anterior pancreaticoduodenal vessels, and along the superior mesenteric vein and right lateral wall of the superior mesenteric artery.

Note

The splenic lymph nodes and those of the tail of the pancreas are not regional; metastases to these lymph nodes are coded M1.

TNM Clinical Classification

T – Primary Tumour

TX	Primary tumour cannot be assessed
T0	No evidence of primary tumour
Tis	Carcinoma in situ

T1a		Tumour limited to ampulla of Vater or sphincter of Oddi
T1b		Tumour invades beyond the sphincter of Oddi (perisphincteric invasion) and/or into the duodenal submucosa
T2		Tumour invades the muscularis propria of the duodenum
T3		Tumour invades pancreas
	T3a	Tumour invades 0.5 cm or less into the pancreas
	T3b	Tumour invades more than 0.5 cm into the pancreas or extends into peripancreatic tissue or duodenal serosa but without involvement of the celiac axis or the superior mesenteric artery

T4 Tumour with vascular involvement of the superior mesenteric artery or celiac axis, or common hepatic artery

N – Regional Lymph Nodes

NX Regional lymph nodes cannot be assessed
N0 No regional lymph node metastasis
N1 Metastasis in 1 or 2 regional lymph nodes
N2 Metastasis in 3 or more regional lymph nodes

M – Distant Metastasis

M0 No distant metastasis
M1 Distant metastasis

pTNM Pathological Classification

The pT and pN categories correspond to the T and N categories. For pM see page 8.

pN0 Histological examination of a regional lymphadenectomy specimen will ordinarily include 12 or more lymph nodes. If the lymph nodes are negative, but the number ordinarily examined is not met, classify as pN0.

Stage – Ampulla of Vater

Stage 0	Tis	N0	M0
Stage IA	T1a	N0	M0
Stage IB	T1b, T2	N0	M0
Stage IIA	T3a	N0	M0
Stage IIB	T3b	N0	M0
Stage IIIA	T1a, T1b, T2, T3	N1	M0
Stage IIIB	Any T	N2	M0
Stage IIIB	T4	Any N	M0
Stage IV	Any T	Any N	M1

Pancreas
(ICD-O-3 C25)

Rules for Classification

The classification applies to carcinomas of the exocrine pancreas and/or high-grade neuroendocrine carcinomas. Well-differentiated neuroendocrine tumours of the pancreas are classified as shown on page 102. There should be histological or cytological confirmation of the disease.

The following are the procedures for assessing T, N, and M categories.

T categories	Physical examination, imaging, and/or surgical exploration
N categories	Physical examination, imaging, and/or surgical exploration
M categories	Physical examination, imaging, and/or surgical exploration

Anatomical Subsites

C25.0	Head of pancreas[a]
C25.1	Body of pancreas[b]
C25.2	Tail of pancreas[c]
C25.3	Pancreatic duct

Notes

[a] Tumours of the head of the pancreas are those arising to the right of the left border of the superior mesenteric vein. The uncinate process is considered as part of the head.

[b] Tumours of the body are those arising between the left border of the superior mesenteric vein and left border of the aorta.

[c] Tumours of the tail are those arising between the left border of the aorta and the hilum of the spleen.

Regional Lymph Nodes

The regional lymph nodes for tumours in the head and neck of the pancreas are the lymph nodes along the common bile duct, common hepatic artery, portal vein, pyloric, infrapyloric, subpyloric, proximal mesenteric, coeliac, posterior, and anterior pancreaticoduodenal vessels, and along the superior mesenteric vein and right lateral wall of the superior mesenteric artery.

The regional lymph nodes for tumours in body and tail are the lymph nodes along the common hepatic artery, coeliac axis, splenic artery, and splenic hilum, as well as retroperitoneal nodes and lateral aortic nodes.

Digestive System

TNM Clinical Classification

T – Primary Tumour

TX   Primary tumour cannot be assessed
T0   No evidence of primary tumour
Tis   Carcinoma in situ*

T1   Tumour 2 cm or less in greatest dimension
      T1a   Tumour 0.5 cm or less in greatest dimension
      T1b   Tumour greater than 0.5 cm and less than 1 cm in greatest dimension
      T1c   Tumour greater than 1 cm but no more than 2 cm in greatest dimension
T2   Tumour more than 2 cm but no more than 4 cm in greatest dimension
T3   Tumour and more than 4 cm in greatest dimension
T4   Tumour involves coeliac axis, superior mesenteric artery and/or common hepatic artery

Note
* Tis also includes the 'PanIN–III' classification.

N – Regional Lymph Nodes

NX   Regional lymph nodes cannot be assessed
N0   No regional lymph node metastasis
N1   Metastases in 1 to 3 regional lymph node
N2   Metastases in 4 or more regional lymph node

M – Distant Metastasis

M0   No distant metastasis
M1   Distant metastasis

pTNM Pathological Classification

The pT and pN categories correspond to the T and N categories. For pM see page 8.

pN0   Histological examination of a regional lymphadenectomy specimen will ordinarily include 12 or more lymph nodes. If the lymph nodes are negative, but the number ordinarily examined is not met, classify as pN0.

Stage – Pancreas

Stage 0	Tis	N0	M0
Stage IA	T1	N0	M0
Stage IB	T2	N0	M0
Stage IIA	T3	N0	M0
Stage IIB	T1, T2, T3	N1	M0
Stage III	T1, T2, T3	N2	M0
	T4	Any N	M0
Stage IV	Any T	Any N	M1

Prognostic Factors Grid – Pancreas

Prognostic risk factors for pancreatic cancer

Prognostic factors	Tumour related	Host related	Environment related
Essential	Distant metastases	ECOG status	Post-resection residual disease or margin status (R0, R1, R2)
Additional	Lymph node metastases CA19-9 level	Postoperative morbidity	Adjuvant therapy
New and promising	hENT1 expression	Modified Glasgow prognostic score (C-reactive protein [CRP] and albumin) Neutrophil-to-lymphocyte ratio (NLR)	Pathological response to neoadjuvant therapy

Digestive System

Source: UICC Manual of Clinical Oncology, Ninth Edition. Edited by Brian O'Sullivan, James D. Brierley, Anil K. D'Cruz, Martin F. Fey, Raphael Pollock, Jan B. Vermorken and Shao Hui Huang. © 2015 UICC. Published 2015 by John Wiley & Sons, Ltd.

Well-Differentiated Neuroendocrine Tumours of the Gastrointestinal Tract

Rules for Classification

This classification system applies to well-differentiated neuroendocrine tumours (carcinoid tumours and atypical carcinoid tumours) of the gastro-intestinal tract, including the pancreas. Neuroendocrine tumours of the lung should be classified according to criteria for carcinoma of the lung. Merkel cell carcinoma of the skin has a separate classification.

High-grade (Grade 3) neuroendocrine carcinomas are excluded and should be classified according to criteria for classifying carcinomas at the respective site.

Histopathological Grading

The following grading scheme has been proposed for all gastrointestinal neuroendocrine tumours:

Grade	Mitotic count (per 10 HPF)[a]	Ki-67 index (%)[b]
G1	<2	≤2
G2	2–20	3–20
G3	>20	>20

Notes
[a] 10 HPF (high power fields) = 2 mm^2; at least 40 fields (at 40× magnification) evaluated in areas of highest mitotic density.
[b] MIB1 antibody; % of 500–2000 tumour cells in areas of highest nuclear labelling.

Well-Differentiated Neuroendocrine Tumours (G1 and G2) – Gastric, Jejunum/Ileum, Appendix, Colonic, and Rectal

Regional lymph nodes

The regional lymph nodes correspond to those listed under the appropriate sites for carcinoma.

TNM Clinical Classification

Stomach

T – Primary Tumour

TX   Primary tumour cannot be assessed
T0   No evidence of primary tumour

T1   Tumour invades lamina propria or submucosa and 1 cm or less in greatest dimension
T2   Tumour invades muscularis propria or is more than 1 cm in greatest dimension
T3   Tumour invades subserosa
T4   Tumour perforates visceral peritoneum (serosa) or invades other organs or adjacent structures

Note
For any T, add (m) for multiple tumours.

N – Regional Lymph Nodes

NX   Regional lymph nodes cannot be assessed
N0   No regional lymph node metastasis
N1   Regional lymph node metastasis

M – Distant Metastasis

M0   No distant metastasis
M1   Distant metastasis
     M1a   Hepatic metastasis(is) only
     M1b   Extrahepatic metastasis(is) only
     M1c   Hepatic and extrahepatic metastases

Stage

Stage I	T1	N0	M0
Stage II	T2, T3	N0	M0
Stage III	T4	N0	M0
	Any T	N1	M0
Stage IV	Any T	Any N	M1

Digestive System

TNM Clinical Classification

Duodenal/Ampullary Tumours

T – Primary Tumour

TX   Primary tumour cannot be assessed
T0   No evidence of primary tumour
T1   Duodenal: Tumour invades mucosa or submucosa and 1 cm or less in greatest dimension
     Ampullary: Tumour 1 cm or less in greatest dimension and confined within the sphincter of Oddi
T2   Duodenal: Tumour invades muscularis propria or is more than 1 cm in greatest dimension
     Ampullary: Tumour invades through sphincter into duodenal submucosa or muscularis propria, or more than 1 cm in greatest dimension
T3   Tumour invades the pancreas or peripancreatic adipose tissue
T4   Tumour perforates visceral peritoneum (serosa) or invades other organs

Note
For any T, add (m) for multiple tumours.

N – Regional Lymph Nodes

NX   Regional lymph nodes cannot be assessed
N0   No regional lymph node metastasis
N1   Regional lymph node metastasis

M – Distant Metastasis

M0   No distant metastasis
M1   Distant metastasis
     M1a   Hepatic metastasis(is) only
     M1b   Extrahepatic metastasis(is) only
     M1c   Hepatic and extrahepatic metastases

Stage

Stage	T	N	M
Stage I	T1	N0	M0
Stage II	T2, T3	N0	M0
Stage III	T4	N0	M0
	Any T	N1	M0
Stage IV	Any T	Any N	M1

TNM Clinical Classification

Jejunum/Ileum

T – Primary Tumour

TX   Primary tumour cannot be assessed
T0   No evidence of primary tumour

T1   Tumour invades lamina propria or submucosa and 1 cm or less in greatest dimension
T2   Tumour invades muscularis propria or is greater than 1 cm in greatest dimension
T3   Tumour invades through the muscularis propria into subserosal tissue without penetration of overlying serosa (jejunal or ileal)
T4   Tumour perforates visceral peritoneum (serosa) or invades other organs or adjacent structures

Note
For any T, add (m) for multiple tumours.

N – Regional Lymph Nodes

NX   Regional lymph nodes cannot be assessed
N0   No regional lymph node metastasis
N1   Less than 12 regional lymph node metastasis without mesenteric mass(es) greater than 2 cm in sizes
N2   12 or more regional nodes and/or mesenteric mass(es) greater than 2 cm in maximum dimension

M – Distant Metastasis

M0   No distant metastasis
M1   Distant metastasis
      M1a   Hepatic metastasis(is) only
      M1b   Extrahepatic metastasis(is) only
      M1c   Hepatic and extrahepatic metastase

Stage

Stage I	T1	N0	M0
Stage II	T2,T3	N0	M0
Stage III	T4	Any N	M0
	Any T	N1, N2	M0
Stage IV	Any T	Any N	M1

Digestive System

TNM Clinical Classification

Appendix

T – Primary Tumour[a]

TX   Primary tumour cannot be assessed
T0   No evidence of primary tumour
T1   Tumour 2 cm or less in greatest dimension
T2   Tumour more than 2 cm but not more than 4 cm in greatest dimension
T3   Tumour more than 4 cm or with subserosal invasion or involvement of the mesoappendix
T4   Tumour perforates peritoneum or invades other adjacent organs or structures, other than direct mural extension to adjacent subserosa, e.g., abdominal wall and skeletal muscle[b]

Notes

[a] High-grade neuroendocrine carcinomas, mixed adenoneuroendocrine carcinomas and goblet cell carcinoid, are excluded and should be classified according to criteria for classifying carcinomas.

[b] Tumour that is adherent to other organs or structures, macroscopically, is classified T4. However, if no tumour is present in the adhesion, microscopically, the classification should be classified pT1–3.

N – Regional Lymph Nodes

NX   Regional lymph nodes cannot be assessed
N0   No regional lymph node metastasis
N1   Regional lymph node metastasis

M – Distant Metastasis

M0   No distant metastasis
M1   Distant metastasis
     M1a   Hepatic metastasis(is) only
     M1b   Extrahepatic metastasis(is) only
     M1c   Hepatic and extrahepatic metastases

pTNM Pathological Classification

The pT and pN categories correspond to the T and N categories. For pM see page 8.

pN0   Histological examination of a regional lymphadenectomy specimen will ordinarily include 12 or more lymph nodes. If the lymph nodes are negative, but the number ordinarily examined is not met, classify as pN0.

Stage

Stage I	T1	N0	M0
Stage II	T2, T3	N0	M0
Stage III	T4	N0	M0
	Any T	N1	M0
Stage IV	Any T	Any N	M1

TNM Clinical Classification

Colon and Rectum

T – Primary Tumour

TX   Primary tumour cannot be assessed
T0   No evidence of primary tumour

T1   Tumour invades lamina propria or submucosa or is no greater than
2 cm in size
   T1a   Tumour less than 1 cm in size
   T1b   Tumour 1 or 2 cm in size
T2   Tumour invades muscularis propria or is greater than 2 cm in size
T3   Tumour invades subserosa, or non-peritonealized pericolic or perirectal
tissues
T4   Tumour perforates the visceral peritoneum or invades other organs

Note
For any T, add (m) for multiple tumours.

N – Regional Lymph Nodes

NX   Regional lymph nodes cannot be assessed
N0   No regional lymph node metastasis
N1   Regional lymph node metastasis

M – Distant Metastasis

M0   No distant metastasis
M1   Distant metastasis
   M1a   Hepatic metastasis(is) only
   M1b   Extrahepatic metastasis(is) only
   M1c   Hepatic and extrahepatic metastases

pTNM Pathological Classification

The pT and pN categories correspond to the T and N categories. For pM see
page 8.

Digestive System

Stage

Stage I	T1	N0	M0
Stage IIA	T2	N0	M0
Stage IIB	T3	N0	M0
Stage IIIA	T4	N0	M0
Stage IIIB	Any T	N1	M0
Stage IV	Any T	Any N	M1

Well-Differentiated Neuroendocrine Tumours – Pancreas (G1 and G2)

Rules for Classification

This classification system applies to well-differentiated neuroendocrine tumours (carcinoid tumours and atypical carcinoid tumours) of the pancreas.

High-grade neuroendocrine carcinomas are excluded and should be classified according to criteria for classifying carcinomas of the pancreas.

Regional lymph nodes

The regional lymph nodes correspond to those listed under the appropriate sites for carcinoma.

TNM Clinical Classification

Pancreas

T – Primary Tumour[a]

TX   Primary tumour cannot be assessed
T0   No evidence of primary tumour

T1   Tumour limited to pancreas,[b] 2 cm or less in greatest dimension
T2   Tumour limited to pancreas[b] more than 2 cm but less than 4 cm in greatest dimension
T3   Tumour limited to pancreas,[b] more than 4 cm in greatest dimension or tumour invading duodenum or bile duct.
T4   Tumour perforates visceral peritoneum (serosa) or invades other organs or adjacent structures

Notes
[a] For any T, add (m) for multiple tumours.
[b] Invasion of adjacent peripancreatic adipose tissue is accepted but invasion of adjacent organs is excluded.

N – Regional Lymph Nodes

NX   Regional lymph nodes cannot be assessed
N0   No regional lymph node metastasis
N1   Regional lymph node metastasis

M – Distant Metastasis

M0   No distant metastasis
M1   Distant metastasis
    M1a   Hepatic metastasis(is) only
    M1b   Extrahepatic metastasis(is) only
    M1c   Hepatic and extrahepatic metastases

Stage

Stage I	T1	N0	M0
Stage II	T2, T3	N0	M0
Stage III	T4	N0	M0
	Any T	N1	M0
Stage IV	Any T	Any N	M1

Digestive System

Lung, Pleural, and Thymic Tumours

Introductory Notes

The classifications apply to carcinomas of the lung including non-small cell and small cell carcinomas, bronchopulmonary carcinoid tumours, malignant mesothelioma of pleura, and thymic tumours.

Each site is described under the following headings:

- Rules for classification with the procedures for assessing T, N, and M categories; additional methods may be used when they enhance the accuracy of appraisal before treatment
- Anatomical subsites where appropriate
- Definition of the regional lymph nodes
- TNM clinical classification
- pTNM pathological classification
- Stage
- Prognostic factors grid

Regional Lymph Nodes

The regional lymph nodes extend from the supraclavicular region to the diaphragm. Direct extension of the primary tumour into lymph nodes is classified as lymph node metastasis.

Lung, Pleural, Thymic

TNM *Classification of Malignant Tumours*, Eighth Edition. Edited by James D. Brierley, Mary K. Gospodarowicz and Christian Wittekind.
© 2017 UICC. Published 2017 by John Wiley & Sons, Ltd.

Lung
(ICD-O-3 C34)

Rules for Classification

The classification applies to carcinomas of the lung including non small cell carcinomas, small cell carcinomas, and bronchopulmonary carcinoid tumours. It does not apply to sarcomas and other rare tumours.

Changes in this edition from the seventh edition are based upon recommendations from the International Association for the Study of Lung Cancer (IASLC) Staging Project (see references).[1-6]

There should be histological confirmation of the disease and division of cases by histological type.

The following are the procedures for assessing T, N, and M categories:

T *categories*   Physical examination, imaging, endoscopy, and/or surgical exploration

N *categories*   Physical examination, imaging, endoscopy, and/or surgical exploration

M *categories*   Physical examination, imaging, and/or surgical exploration

Anatomical Subsites

1. Main bronchus (C34.0)
2. Upper lobe (C34.1)
3. Middle lobe (C34.2)
4. Lower lobe (C34.3)

Regional Lymph Nodes

The regional lymph nodes are the intrathoracic nodes (mediastinal, hilar, lobar, interlobar, segmental, and subsegmental), scalene, and supraclavicular lymph nodes.

TNM Clinical Classification

T – Primary Tumour

TX   Primary tumour cannot be assessed, or tumour proven by the presence of malignant cells in sputum or bronchial washings but not visualized by imaging or bronchoscopy

T0   No evidence of primary tumour
Tis Carcinoma in situ[a]

T1   Tumour 3 cm or less in greatest dimension, surrounded by lung or visceral pleura, without bronchoscopic evidence of invasion more proximal than the lobar bronchus (i.e., not in the main bronchus)[b]

T1mi   Minimally invasive adenocarcinoma[c]
T1a   Tumour 1 cm or less in greatest dimension[b]
T1b   Tumour more than 1 cm but not more than 2 cm in greatest dimension[b]
T1c   Tumour more than 2 cm but not more than 3 cm in greatest dimension[b]

T2   Tumour more than 3 cm but not more than 5 cm; or tumour with *any* of the following features[d]
  - Involves main bronchus regardless of distance to the carina, but without involvement of the carina
  - Invades visceral pleura
  - Associated with atelectasis or obstructive pneumonitis that extends to the hilar region either involving part of or the entire lung

T2a   Tumour more than 3 cm but not more than 4 cm in greatest dimension
T2b   Tumour more than 4 cm but not more than 5 cm in greatest dimension

T3   Tumour more than 5 cm but not more than 7 cm in greatest dimension or one that directly invades any of the following: parietal pleura, chest wall (including superior sulcus tumours) phrenic nerve, parietal pericardium; or separate tumour nodule(s) in the same lobe as the primary

T4   Tumour more than 7 cm or of any size that invades any of the following: diaphragm, mediastinum, heart, great vessels, trachea, recurrent laryngeal nerve, oesophagus, vertebral body, carina; separate tumour nodule(s) in a different ipsilateral lobe to that of the primary

N – Regional Lymph Nodes

NX   Regional lymph nodes cannot be assessed
N0   No regional lymph node metastasis
N1   Metastasis in ipsilateral peribronchial and/or ipsilateral hilar lymph nodes and intrapulmonary nodes, including involvement by direct extension

Lung, Pleural, Thymic

N2 Metastasis in ipsilateral mediastinal and/or subcarinal lymph node(s)

N3 Metastasis in contralateral mediastinal, contralateral hilar, ipsilateral or contralateral scalene, or supraclavicular lymph node(s)

M – Distant Metastasis

M0 No distant metastasis

M1 Distant metastasis

M1a Separate tumour nodule(s) in a contralateral lobe; tumour with pleural or pericardial nodules or malignant pleural or pericardial effusion[e]

M1b Single extrathoracic metastasis in a single organ[f]

M1c Multiple extrathoracic metastasis in a single or multiple organs

Notes

[a] Tis includes adenocarcinoma in situ and squamous carcinoma in situ.

[b] The uncommon superficial spreading tumour of any size with its invasive component limited to the bronchial wall, which may extend proximal to the main bronchus, is also classified as T1a.

[c] Solitary adenocarcinoma (not more than 3 cm in greatest dimension), with a predominantly lepidic pattern and not more than 5 mm invasion in greatest dimension in any one focus.

[d] T2 tumours with these features are classified T2a if 4 cm or less, or if size cannot be determined and T2b if greater than 4 cm but not larger than 5 cm.

[e] Most pleural (pericardial) effusions with lung cancer are due to tumour. In a few patients, however, multiple microscopic examinations of pleural (pericardial) fluid are negative for tumour, and the fluid is non-bloody and is not an exudate. Where these elements and clinical judgment dictate that the effusion is not related to the tumour, the effusion should be excluded as a staging descriptor.

[f] This includes involvement of a single non-regional node.

pTNM Pathological Classification

The pT and pN categories correspond to the T and N categories. For pM see page 8.

pN0 Histological examination of hilar and mediastinal lymphadenectomy specimen(s) will ordinarily include 6 or more lymph nodes/stations. Three of these nodes/stations should be mediastinal, including the subcarinal nodes and three from N1 nodes/stations. Labelling according to the IASLC chart and table of definitions given in the TNM Supplement is desirable. If all the lymph nodes examined are negative, but the number ordinarily examined is not met, classify as pN0.

Stage

Occult carcinoma	TX	N0	M0
Stage 0	Tis	N0	M0
Stage IA	T1	N0	M0
Stage IA1	T1mi	N0	M0
	T1a	N0	M0
Stage IA2	T1b	N0	M0
Stage IA3	T1c	N0	M0
Stage IB	T2a	N0	M0
Stage IIA	T2b	N0	M0
Stage IIB	T1a-c, T2a,b	N1	M0
	T3	N0	M0
Stage IIIA	T1a-c, T2a,b	N2	M0
	T3	N1,	M0
	T4	N0, N1	M0
Stage IIIB	T1a-c, T2a,b	N3	M0
	T3, T4	N2	M0
Stage IIIC	T3, T4	N3	M0
Stage IV	Any T	Any N	M1
Stage IVA	Any T	Any N	M1a, M1b
Stage IVB	Any T	Any N	M1c

Prognostic Factors Grid – Non-Small Cell Lung Carcinoma

Prognostic factors in surgically resected NSCLC

Prognostic factors	Tumour related	Host related	Environment related
Essential	T category N category Extracapsular nodal extension	Weight loss Performance status	Resection margins Adequacy of mediastinal dissection
Additional	Histological type Grade Vessel invasion Tumour size	Gender	
New and promising	Molecular/ biological markers	Quality of life Marital status	

Prognostic risk factors in advanced (locally-advanced or metastatic) NSCLC

Prognostic factors	Tumour related	Host related	Environment related
Essential	Stage Superior vena cava obstruction (SVCO) Oligometastatic disease Number of sites	Weight loss Performance status	Chemotherapy Targeted therapy
Additional	Number of metastatic sites Pleural effusion Liver metastasis Haemoglobin Lactate dehydrogenase (LDH) Albumin	Gender Symptom burden	
New and promising	Molecular/biological markers	Quality of life Marital status Anxiety/ depression	

Source: UICC Manual of Clinical Oncology, Ninth Edition. Edited by Brian O'Sullivan, James D. Brierley, Anil K. D'Cruz, Martin F. Fey, Raphael Pollock, Jan B. Vermorken and Shao Hui Huang. © 2015 UICC. Published 2015 by John Wiley & Sons, Ltd.

Prognostic Factors Grid – Small Cell Lung Carcinoma

Prognostic risk factors in SCLC

Prognostic factors	Tumour related	Host related	Environment related
Essential	Stage	Performance status Age Comorbidity	Chemotherapy Thoracic radiotherapy Prophylactic cranial radiotherapy
Additional	LDH		
	Alkaline phosphatase Cushing syndrome M0 – mediastinal involvement M1 – number of sites Brain or bone involvement White blood cell count (WBC)/platelet count		
New and promising	Molecular/biological markers		

Source: UICC Manual of Clinical Oncology, Ninth Edition. Edited by Brian O'Sullivan, James D. Brierley, Anil K. D'Cruz, Martin F. Fey, Raphael Pollock, Jan B. Vermorken and Shao Hui Huang. © 2015 UICC. Published 2015 by John Wiley & Sons, Ltd.

References

1 Rami-Porta R, Bolejack V, Giroux DJ, et al. The IASLC Lung Cancer Staging Project: the new database to inform the 8th edition of the TNM classification of lung cancer. J Thorac Oncol 2014; 9: 1618–1624.

2 Rami-Porta R, Bolejack V, Crowley J, et al. The IASLC Lung Cancer Staging Project: proposals for the revisions of the T descriptors in the forthcoming 8th edition of the TNM classification for lung cancer. J Thorac Oncol 2015; 10: 990–1003.

3 Asamura H, Chansky K, Crowley J, et al. The IASLC Lung Cancer Staging Project: proposals for the revisions of the N descriptors in the forthcoming 8th edition of the TNM classification for lung cancer. J Thorac Oncol 2015; 10: 1675–1684.

4 Eberhardt WEE, Mitchell A, Crowley J, et al. The IASLC Lung Cancer Staging Project: proposals for the revisions of the M descriptors in the forthcoming 8th edition of the TNM classification for lung cancer. J Thorac Oncol 2015; 10: 1515–1522.

5 Goldstraw P et al. The IASLC Lung Cancer Staging Project: proposals for the revision of the TNM stage grouping in the forthcoming (eighth) edition of the TNM classification for lung cancer. *J Thorac Oncol* 2016;11: 39–51.

6 Nicholson AG, Chansky K, Crowley J, et al. The IASLC Lung Cancer Staging Project: proposals for the revision of the clinical and pathological staging of small cell lung cancer in the forthcoming eighth edition of the TNM classification for lung cancer. *J Thorac Oncol* 2016;11: 300–311.

Pleural Mesothelioma
(ICD-O C38.4)

Rules for Classification

The classification applies only to malignant mesothelioma of the pleura. There should be histological confirmation of the disease.

Changes in this edition from the seventh edition are based upon recommendations from the International Association for the Study of Lung Cancer (IASLC) Staging Project.

The following are the procedures for assessing T, N, and M categories:

T *categories*	Physical examination, imaging, endoscopy, and/or surgical exploration
N *categories*	Physical examination, imaging, endoscopy, and/or surgical exploration
M *categories*	Physical examination, imaging, and/or surgical exploration

Regional Lymph Nodes

The regional lymph nodes are the intrathoracic, internal mammary, scalene, and supraclavicular nodes.

TNM Clinical Classification

T – Primary Tumour

TX Primary tumour cannot be assessed
T0 No evidence of primary tumour

T1 Tumour involves ipsilateral parietal or visceral pleura only, with or without involvement of visceral, mediastinal or diaphragmatic pleura.

T2 Tumour involves the ipsilateral pleura (parietal or visceral pleura), with at least one of the following:
  - invasion of diaphragmatic muscle
  - invasion of lung parenchyma

T3 Tumour involves ipsilateral pleura (parietal or visceral pleura), with at least one of the following:
  - invasion of endothoracic fascia
  - invasion into mediastinal fat
  - solitary focus of tumour invading soft tissues of the chest wall
  - non-transmural involvement of the pericardium

Lung, Pleural, Thymic

T4 Tumour involves ipsilateral pleura (parietal or visceral pleura), with at least one of the following:
- chest wall, with or without associated rib destruction (diffuse or multifocal)
- peritoneum (via direct transdiaphragmatic extension)
- contralateral pleura
- mediastinal organs (oesophagus, trachea, heart, great vessels)
- vertebra, neuroforamen, spinal cord
- internal surface of the pericardium (transmural invasion with or without a pericardial effusion)

N – Regional Lymph Nodes

NX Regional lymph nodes cannot be assessed
N0 No regional lymph node metastasis
N1 Metastases to ipsilateral intrathoracic lymph nodes (includes ipsilateral bronchopulmonary, hilar, subcarinal, paratracheal, aortopulmonary, paraesophageal, peridiaphragmatic, pericardial fat pad, intercostal and internal mammary nodes)
N2 Metastases to contralateral intrathoracic lymph nodes. Metastases to ipsilateral or contralateral supraclavicular lymph nodes

M – Distant Metastasis

M0 No distant metastasis
M1 Distant metastasis

pTNM Pathological Classification

The pT and pN categories correspond to the T and N categories. For pM see page 8.

Stage – Pleural Mesothelioma

Stage IA	T1	N0	M0
Stage IB	T2,T3	N0	M0
Stage II	T1,T2	N1	M0
Stage IIIA	T3	N1	M0
Stage IIIB	T1,T2,T3	N2	M0
	T4	Any N	M0
Stage IV	Any T	Any N	M1

Thymic Tumours
ICD-O-3 C37.9

Rules for Classification

The classification applies to epithelial tumours of the thymus, including thymomas, thymic carcinomas and neuroendocrine tumours of the thymus. It does not apply to sarcomas, lymphomas and other rare tumours.

This classification is new to the 8th edition and is based upon recommendations from the International Association for the Study of Lung Cancer (IASLC) Staging Project and the International Thymic Malignancies Interest Group (ITMIG) (see references).[1–3]

There should be histological confirmation of the disease and division of cases by histological type.

The following are the procedures for assessing T, N, and M categories:

T categories   Physical examination, imaging, endoscopy, and/or surgical exploration

N categories   Physical examination, imaging, endoscopy, and/or surgical exploration

M categories   Physical examination, imaging, and/or surgical exploration

Regional Lymph Nodes

The regional lymph nodes are the anterior (perithymic) lymph nodes, the deep intrathoracic lymph nodes and the cervical lymph nodes.

TNM Clinical Classification

T – Primary Tumour

TX   Primary tumour cannot be assessed
T0   No evidence of primary tumour

T1   Tumour encapsulated or extending into the mediastinal fat, may involve the mediastinal pleura.
   T1a   No mediastinal pleural involvement
   T1b   Direct invasion of the mediastinal pleura
T2   Tumour with direct involvement of the pericardium (partial or full thickness).
T3   Tumour with direct invasion into any of the following; lung, brachiocephalic vein, superior vena cava, phrenic nerve, chest wall, or extrapericardial pulmonary artery or vein.

T4   Tumour with direct invasion into any of the following; aorta (ascending, arch or descending), arch vessels, intrapericardial pulmonary artery, myocardium, trachea, or oesophagus

N – Regional Lymph Nodes

NX   Regional lymph nodes cannot be assessed
N0   No regional lymph node metastasis
N1   Metastasis in anterior (perithymic) lymph nodes
N2   Metastasis in deep intrathoracic or cervical lymph nodes

M – Distant Metastasis

M0   No pleural, pericardial or distant metastasis
M1   Distant metastasis
    M1a   Separate pleural or pericardial nodule(s)
    M1b   Distant metastasis beyond the pleura or pericardium

TNM Pathological Classification

The pT and pN categories correspond to the T and N categories. For pM see page 8.

Stage –THYMUS TUMOURS

Stage	T	N	M
Stage I	T1	N0	M0
Stage II	T2	N0	M0
Stage IIIA	T3	N0	M0
Stage IIIB	T4	N0	M0
Stage IVA	Any T	N1	M0
	Any T	N0, N1	M1a
Stage IVB	Any T	N2	M0, M1a
	Any T	Any N	M1b

References

1 Nicholson AG, Detterbeck FC, Marino M, et al. The IASLC/ITMIG thymic epithelial tumors staging project: proposals for the T component for the forthcoming (8th) edition of the TNM classification of malignant tumors. *J Thorac Oncol* 2014; 9: s73–s80.

2 Kondo K, Van Schil P, Detterbeck FC, et al. The IASLC/ITMIG thymic epithelial tumors staging project: proposals for the N and M components for the forthcoming (8th) edition of the TNM classification of malignant tumors. J *Thorac Oncol* 2014; 9: s81–s87.

3 Detterbeck FC, Stratton K, Giroux D, et al. The IASLC/ITMIG thymic epithelial tumors staging project: proposal for an evidence-based stage classification system for the forthcoming (8th) edition of the TNM classification of malignant tumors. J *Thorac Oncol* 2014; 9: s65–s72.

Tumours of Bone and Soft Tissues

Introductory Notes

The following sites are included:
- Bone
- Soft tissues
- Gastrointestinal stromal tumours

Each site is described under the following headings:
- Rules for classification with the procedures for assessing T, N, and M categories; additional methods may be used when they enhance the accuracy of appraisal before treatment
- Anatomical sites where appropriate
- Definition of the regional lymph nodes
- TNM clinical classification
- pTNM pathological classification
- G histopathological grading
- Stage
- Prognostic factors grid

G Histopathological Grading

The staging of bone and soft tissue sarcomas is based on a three-tiered grade classification. In this classification, Grade 1 is considered 'low grade' and Grades 2 and 3 'high grade'.

TNM Classification of Malignant Tumours, Eighth Edition. Edited by James D. Brierley, Mary K. Gospodarowicz and Christian Wittekind.
© 2017 UICC. Published 2017 by John Wiley & Sons, Ltd.

Bone
(ICD-O-3 C40, 41)

Rules for Classification

The classification applies to all primary malignant bone tumours except malignant lymphoma, multiple myeloma, surface/juxtacortical osteosarcoma, and juxtacortical chondrosarcoma. There should be histological confirmation of the disease and division of cases by histological type and grade.

The following are the procedures for assessing T, N, and M categories:

T categories	Physical examination and imaging
N categories	Physical examination and imaging
M categories	Physical examination and imaging

Regional Lymph Nodes

The regional lymph nodes are those appropriate to the site of the primary tumour. Regional node involvement is rare and cases in which nodal status is not assessed either clinically or pathologically could be considered N0 instead of NX or pNX.

TNM Clinical Classification

T – Primary Tumour

TX Primary tumour cannot be assessed
T0 No evidence of primary tumour

Appendicular Skeleton, Trunk, Skull and Facial Bones

T1 Tumour 8 cm or less in greatest dimension
T2 Tumour more than 8 cm in greatest dimension
T3 Discontinuous tumours in the primary bone site

Spine

T1 Tumour confined to a single vertebral segment or two adjacent vertebral segments
T2 Tumour confined to three adjacent vertebral segments

T3   Tumour confined to four adjacent vertebral segments

T4a   Tumour invades into the spinal canal

T4b   Tumour invades the adjacent vessels or tumour thrombosis within the adjacent vessels

Note

The five vertebral segments are the:

    Right pedicle

    Right body

    Left body

    Left pedicle

    Posterior element

Pelvis

T1a   A tumour 8 cm or less in size and confined to a single pelvic segment with no extraosseous extension

T1b   A tumour greater than 8 cm in size and confined to a single pelvic segment with no extraosseous extension

T2a   A tumour 8 cm or less in size and confined to a single pelvic segment with extraosseous extension or confined to two adjacent pelvic segments without extraosseous extension

T2b   A tumour greater than 8 cm in size and confined to a single pelvic segment with extraosseous extension or confined to two adjacent pelvic segments without extraosseous extension

T3a   A tumour 8 cm or less in size and confined to two pelvic segments with extraosseous extension

T3b   A tumour greater than 8 cm in size and confined to two pelvic segment with extraosseous extension

T4a   Tumour involving three adjacent pelvic segments or crossing the sacroiliac joint to the sacral neuroforamen

T4b   Tumour encasing the external iliac vessels or gross tumour thrombus in major pelvic vessels

Note

The four pelvic segments are the:

    Sacrum lateral to the sacral foramen,

    Iliac wing,

    Acetabulum/periacetabulum and

    Pelvic rami, symphysis and ischium

N – Regional Lymph Nodes

NX   Regional lymph nodes cannot be assessed
N0   No regional lymph node metastasis
N1   Regional lymph node metastasis

M – Distant Metastasis

M0   No distant metastasis
M1   Distant metastasis
     M1a   Lung
     M1b   Other distant sites

pTNM Pathological Classification

The pT and pN categories correspond to the T and N categories. For pM see page 8.

Stage – Appendicular Skeleton, Trunk, Skull and Facial Bones

Stage IA	T1	N0	M0	G1, GX Low Grade
Stage IB	T2, T3	N0	M0	G1, GX Low Grade
Stage IIA	T1	N0	M0	G2, G3 High Grade
Stage IIB	T2	N0	M0	G2, G3 High Grade
Stage III	T3	N0	M0	G2, G3 High Grade
Stage IVA	Any T	N0	M1a	Any G
Stage IVB	Any T	N1	Any M	Any G
Stage IVB	Any T	N0	M1b	Any G

Stage – Spine and Pelvis

There is no stage for bone sarcomas of the spine or pelvis.

Prognostic Factors Grid – Bone

Prognostic factors for osteosarcoma

Prognostic factors	Tumour related	Host related	Environment related
Essential	Location, size, extent of disease Tumour response to neoadjuvant chemotherapy	Age	Residual disease after resection
Additional	LDH Alkaline phosphatase	Gender Performance status	Management by a multidisciplinary sarcoma team Local recurrence
New and promising	Biomarkers		

Source: UICC Manual of Clinical Oncology, Ninth Edition. Edited by Brian O'Sullivan, James D. Brierley, Anil K. D'Cruz, Martin F. Fey, Raphael Pollock, Jan B. Vermorken and Shao Hui Huang. © 2015 UICC. Published 2015 by John Wiley & Sons, Ltd.

Soft Tissues
(ICD-O-3 C38.1, 2, C47-49)

Rules for Classification

There should be histological confirmation of the disease and division of cases by histological type and grade.

The following are the procedures for assessing T, N, and M categories:

T *categories*   Physical examination and imaging
N *categories*   Physical examination and imaging
M *categories*   Physical examination and imaging

Anatomical Sites

1. Connective, subcutaneous, and other soft tissues (C49), peripheral nerves (C47)
2. Retroperitoneum (C48.0)
3. Mediastinum: anterior (C38.1); posterior (C38.2); mediastinum, NOS (C38.3)

Histological Types of Tumour

The following histological types are not included:
- Kaposi sarcoma
- Dermatofibrosarcoma (protuberans)
- Fibromatosis (desmoid tumour)
- Sarcoma arising from the dura mater, brain, hollow viscera, or paren-chymatous organs (with the exception of breast sarcomas)
- Angiosarcoma, an aggressive sarcoma, is excluded because its natural history is not consistent with the classification.

Regional Lymph Nodes

The regional lymph nodes are those appropriate to the site of the primary tumour. Regional node involvement is rare and cases in which nodal status is not assessed either clinically or pathologically could be considered N0 instead of NX or pNX.

TNM Clinical Classification

T – Primary Tumour

TX   Primary tumour cannot be assessed
T0   No evidence of primary tumour

Extremity and Superficial Trunk

T1   Tumour 5 cm or less in greatest dimension
T2   Tumour more than 5 cm but no more than 10 cm in greatest dimension
T3   Tumour more than 10 cm but no more than 15 cm in greatest dimension
T4   Tumour more than 15 cm in greatest dimension

Retroperitoneum

T1   Tumour 5 cm or less in greatest dimension
T2   Tumour more than 5 cm but no more than 10 cm in greatest dimension
T3   Tumour more than 10 cm but no more than 15 cm in greatest dimension
T4   Tumour more than 15 cm in greatest dimension

Head and Neck

T1   Tumour 2 cm or less in greatest dimension
T2   Tumour more than 2 cm but no more than 4 cm in greatest
T3   Tumour more than 4 cm in greatest dimension
T4a Tumour invades the orbit, skull base or dura, central compartment viscera, facial skeleton, and or pterygoid muscles
T4b Tumour invades the brain parenchyma, encases the carotid artery, invades prevertebral muscle or involves the central nervous system by perineural spread

Thoracic and Abdominal Viscera

T1   Tumour confined to a single organ
T2a Tumour invades serosa or visceral peritoneum
T2b Tumour with microscopic extension beyond the serosa
T3   Tumour invades another organ or macroscopic extension beyond the serosa

T4a	Multifocal tumour involving no more than two sites in one organ
T4b	Multifocal tumour involving more than two sites but not more then 5 sites
T4c	Multifocal tumour involving more than five sites

N – Regional Lymph Nodes

NX	Regional lymph nodes cannot be assessed
N0	No regional lymph node metastasis
N1	Regional lymph node metastasis

M – Distant Metastasis

| M0 | No distant metastasis |
| M1 | Distant metastasis |

pTNM Pathological Classification

The pT and pN categories correspond to the T and N categories. For pM see page 8.

Stage – Extremity and Superficial Trunk and Retroperitoneum

Stage IA	T1	N0	M0	G1, GX Low Grade
Stage IB	T2, T3, T4	N0	M0	G1, GX Low Grade
Stage II	T1	N0	M0	G2, G3 High Grade
Stage IIIA	T2	N0	M0	G2, G3 High Grade
Stage IIIB	T3, T4	N0	M0	G2, G3 High Grade
Stage IIIB	Any T	N1*	M0	Any G
Stage IV	Any T	Any N	M1	Any G

Note

* AJCC classifies N1 as stage IV for extremity and superficial trunk.

Stage – Head and Neck and Thoracic and Abdominal Viscera

There is no stage for soft tissue sarcoma of the head and neck and thoracic and abdominal viscera.

Gastrointestinal Stromal Tumour (GIST)

Rules for Classification

The classification applies only to gastrointestinal stromal tumours. There should be histological confirmation of the disease.

The following are the procedures for assessing the T, N, and M categories.

T *categories*	Physical examination, imaging, endoscopy, and/or surgical exploration
N *categories*	Physical examination, imaging, and/or surgical exploration
M *categories*	Physical examination, imaging, and/or surgical exploration

Anatomical Sites and Subsites

- Oesophagus (C15)
- Stomach (C16)
- Small intestine (C17)
  1. Duodenum (C17.0)
  2. Jejunum (C17.1)
  3. Ileum (C17.2)
- Colon (C18)
- Rectum (C20)
- Omentum (C48.1)
- Mesentery (C48.1)

Regional Lymph Nodes

The regional lymph nodes are those appropriate to the site of the primary tumour; see gastrointestinal sites for details.

TNM Clinical Classification

T – Primary Tumour

TX   Primary tumour cannot be assessed
T0   No evidence for primary tumour

T1   Tumour 2 cm or less
T2   Tumour more than 2 cm but not more than 5 cm
T3   Tumour more than 5 cm but not more than 10 cm
T4   Tumour more than 10 cm in greatest dimension

N – Regional Lymph Nodes

NX   Regional lymph nodes cannot be assessed*
N0   No regional lymph node metastasis
N1   Regional lymph node metastasis

Note
*NX: Regional lymph node involvement is rare for GISTs, so that cases in which the nodal status is not assessed clinically or pathologically could be considered N0 instead of NX or pNX.

M – Distant Metastasis

M0   No distant metastasis
M1   Distant metastasis

pTNM Pathological Classification

The pT and pN categories correspond to the T and N categories. For pM see page 8.

G Histopathological Grading

Grading for GIST is dependent on mitotic rate.*
Low mitotic rate: 5 or fewer per 50 hpf
High mitotic rate: over 5 per 50 hpf

Note
* The mitotic rate of GIST is best expressed as the number of mitoses per 50 high power fields (hpf) using the 40× objective (total area 5 mm^2 in 50 fields).

Stage

Staging criteria for gastric tumours can be applied in primary, solitary omental GISTs. Staging criteria for intestinal tumours can be applied to GISTs in less common sites such as oesophagus, colon, rectum, and mesentery.

Gastric GIST

				Mitotic rate
Stage IA	T1, T2	N0	M0	Low
Stage IB	T3	N0	M0	Low
Stage II	T1, T2	N0	M0	High
	T4	N0	M0	Low
Stage IIIA	T3	N0	M0	High
Stage IIIB	T4	N0	M0	High
Stage IV	Any T	N1	M0	Any rate
	Any T	Any N	M1	Any rate

Small Intestinal GIST

				Mitotic rate
Stage I	T1, T2	N0	M0	Low
Stage II	T3	N0	M0	Low
Stage IIIA	T1	N0	M0	High
	T4	N0	M0	Low
Stage IIIB	T2, T3, T4	N0	M0	High
Stage IV	Any T	N1	M0	Any rate
	Any T	Any N	M1	Any rate

Bone & Soft Tissues

Prognostic Factor Grid – Soft Tissue Sarcoma and GIST

Prognostic factors for soft tissue sarcomas

Prognostic factors	Tumour related	Host related	Environment related
Essential	Anatomical site Histological type Size of tumour: • < or >5 cm in general • ≤2, 2–≤5, 5–≤10 and >10 cm for GIST Depth of invasion Grade (well to poorly differentiated) M category Mitotic rate for GIST (<5 mitoses and ≥5 mitoses/50 HPF)		
Additional	Presence of *c*-Kit mutation for GIST Mutational site in *c*-Kit or *PDGFRA* gene for GIST *EWS–FL11* fusion transcript for Ewing sarcoma *SYT–SSX* fusion transcript for synovial sarcoma *FOXO1* translocation for alveolar rhabdomyosarcoma Surgical resection margins Presentation status (primary vs recurrence)	Neurofi-bromatosis (NF1) Radiation-induced sarcomas Age	Quality of surgery and radiotherapy
New and promising	TP53 Ki-67 Tumour hypoxia		

Source: UICC Manual of Clinical Oncology, Ninth Edition. Edited by Brian O'Sullivan, James D. Brierley, Anil K. D'Cruz, Martin F. Fey, Raphael Pollock, Jan B. Vermorken and Shao Hui Huang. © 2015 UICC. Published 2015 by John Wiley & Sons, Ltd.

Skin Tumours

Introductory Notes

The classifications apply to: carcinomas of the skin,* [excluding vulva (see page 161), penis (see page 188), and perianal skin (see page 77)], malignant melanomas of the skin including eyelid, and to Merkel cell carcinoma.

Note
* There is a new classification for carcinoma of the skin of the head and neck region.

Anatomical Sites

The following sites are identified by ICD-O-3 topography rubrics:
- Lip (excluding vermilion surface) (C44.0)
- Eyelid (C44.1)
- External ear (C44.2)
- Other and unspecified parts of face (C44.3)
- Scalp and neck (C44.4)
- Trunk excluding anal margin and perianal skin (C44.5)
- Upper limb and shoulder (C44.6)
- Lower limb and hip (C44.7)
- Scrotum (C63.2)

Each tumour type is described under the following headings:
- Rules for classification with the procedures for assessing T, N, and M categories
- Regional lymph nodes
- TNM clinical classification
- pTNM pathological classification
- Stage
- Prognostic factors grid

TNM Classification of Malignant Tumours, Eighth Edition. Edited by James D. Brierley, Mary K. Gospodarowicz and Christian Wittekind.
© 2017 UICC. Published 2017 by John Wiley & Sons, Ltd.

Regional Lymph Nodes

The regional lymph nodes are those appropriate to the site of the primary tumour.

Unilateral Tumours

- **Head, neck:** Ipsilateral preauricular, submandibular, cervical, and supraclavicular lymph nodes
- **Thorax:** Ipsilateral axillary lymph nodes
- **Upper limb:** Ipsilateral epitrochlear and axillary lymph nodes
- **Abdomen, loins, and buttocks:** Ipsilateral inguinal lymph nodes
- **Lower limb:** Ipsilateral popliteal and inguinal lymph nodes

Tumours in the Boundary Zones Between these sites

The lymph nodes pertaining to the regions on both sides of the boundary zone are considered to be the regional lymph nodes.

The following 4-cm wide bands are considered as boundary zones:

Between	Along
Right/left	Midline
Head and neck/thorax	Clavicula–acromion–upper shoulder blade edge
Thorax/upper limb	Shoulder–axilla–shoulder
Thorax/abdomen, loins, and buttocks	*Front*: middle between navel and costal arch
	Back: lower border of thoracic vertebrae (midtransverse axis)
Abdomen, loins, and buttock/lower limb	Groin–trochanter–gluteal Sulcus

Any metastasis to other than the listed regional lymph nodes is considered as M1.

Carcinoma of Skin (excluding eyelid, head and neck, perianal, vulva, and penis) (ICD-O-3 C44.5-7, C63.2)*

Rules for Classification*

The classification applies only to carcinomas, excluding Merkel cell carcinoma. There should be histological confirmation of the disease and division of cases by histological type.

The following are the procedures for assessing T, N, and M categories:

T categories   Physical examination
N categories   Physical examination and imaging
M categories   Physical examination and imaging

Note
* The AJCC only includes the classification for skin carcinoma of the head and neck.

Regional Lymph Nodes

The regional lymph nodes are those appropriate to the site of the primary tumour. See page 132.

TNM Clinical Classification

T – Primary Tumour

TX   Primary tumour cannot be identified
T0   No evidence of primary tumour
Tis   Carcinoma in situ

T1   Tumour 2 cm or less in greatest dimension
T2   Tumour >2 cm and ≤4 cm in greatest dimension
T3   Tumour >4 cm in greatest dimension or minor bone erosion or perineural invasion or deep invasion*
T4a   Tumour with gross cortical bone/marrow invasion
T4b   Tumour with axial skeleton invasion including foraminal involvement and/or vertebral foramen involvement to the epidural space

Note
* Deep invasion is defined as invasion beyond the subcutaneous fat or >6 mm (as measured from the granular layer of adjacent normal epidermis to the base of the tumour);

perineural invasion forT3 classification is defined as clinical or radiographic involvement of named nerves without foramen or skull base invasion or transgression.

In the case of multiple simultaneous tumours, the tumour with the highest T category is classified and the number of separate tumours is indicated in parentheses, e.g., T2(5).

N – Regional Lymph Nodes

NX   Regional lymph nodes cannot be assessed
N0   No regional lymph node metastasis
N1   Metastasis in a single lymph node 3 cm or less in greatest dimension
N2   Metastasis in a single ipsilateral lymph node, more than 3 cm but not more than 6 cm in greatest dimension or in multiple ipsilateral nodes none more than 6 cm in greatest dimension
N3   Metastasis in a lymph node more than 6 cm in greatest dimension

M – Distant Metastasis

M0   No distant metastasis
M1   Distant metastatic disease*

Note
* Contralateral nodes in non-melanoma non-head and neck cancer are distant metastases.

pTNM Pathological Classification

The pT and pN categories correspond to the T and N categories. For pM see page 8.

pN0   Histological examination of a regional lymphadenectomy specimen will ordinarily include 6 or more lymph nodes. If the lymph nodes are negative, but the number ordinarily examined is not met, classify as pN0.

Stage

Stage 0	Tis	N0	M0
Stage I	T1	N0	M0
Stage II	T2	N0	M0
Stage III	T3	N0	M0
	T1, T2, T3	N1	M0

Stage IVA	T1, T2, T3	N2, N3	M0
	T4	Any N	M0
Stage IVB	Any T	Any N	M1

Prognostic Factors Grid – Non-Melanoma Skin

Tumour-, host- and environment-related prognostic factors
for skin cancer

Prognostic factors	Tumour related	Host related	Environment related
Essential	TNM Histopathological type Location Thickness PNI (clinical)	Immune suppression Recurrent disease	Surgical margins Previous RT
Additional	Tumour borders Differentiation Rate of growth LVSI PNI (incidental)	Genetic factors Gorlin syndrome Age Chronic inflammation, scars, burns	Smoking (SCC)
New and promising	SLNB Perturbed cellular pathways		Viral aetiology Highly conformal RT Chemoradiotherapy Targeted therapies Intralesional therapy

Skin

Source: UICC Manual of Clinical Oncology, Ninth Edition. Edited by Brian O'Sullivan, James D. Brierley, Anil K. D'Cruz, Martin F. Fey, Raphael Pollock, Jan B. Vermorken and Shao Hui Huang. © 2015 UICC. Published 2015 by John Wiley & Sons, Ltd.

Skin Carcinoma of the Head and Neck (ICD-O-3 C44.0 C44.2-4)

Rules for Classification

The classification applies only to cutaneous carcinomas of the head and neck region excluding the eyelid and excluding Merkel cell carcinoma and malignant melanoma. There should be histological confirmation of the disease.

The following are the procedures for assessing T, N, and M categories:

T categories	Physical examination and imaging
N categories	Physical examination and imaging
M categories	Physical examination and imaging

Anatomical Sites

The following sites are identified by ICD-O topography rubrics:
- Lip (excluding vermilion surface) (C44.0)
- External ear (C44.2)
- Other and unspecified parts of face (C44.3)
- Scalp and neck (C44.4)

TNM Clinical Classification

T – Primary Tumour

TX   Primary tumour cannot be identified
T0   No evidence of primary tumour
Tis   Carcinoma in situ

T1   Tumour 2 cm or less in greatest dimension
T2   Tumour >2 cm and ≤4 cm in greatest dimension
T3   Tumour >4 cm in greatest dimension or minor bone erosion or perineural invasion or deep invasion*
T4a   Tumour with gross cortical bone/marrow invasion
T4b   Tumour with skull base or axial skeleton invasion including foraminal involvement and/or vertebral foramen involvement to the epidural space

Note

* Deep invasion is defined as invasion beyond the subcutaneous fat or >6 mm (as measured from the granular layer of adjacent normal epidermis to the base of the tumour), perineural invasion for T3 classification is defined as clinical or radiographic involvement of named nerves without foramen or skull base invasion or transgression.

N – Regional Lymph Nodes

N0   No regional lymph node metastasis

N1   Metastasis in a single ipsilateral lymph node, 3 cm or less in greatest dimension without extranodal extension

N2   Metastasis described as:

    N2a   Metastasis in a single ipsilateral lymph node more than 3 cm but not more than 6 cm in greatest dimension without extranodal extension

    N2b   Metastasis in multiple ipsilateral lymph nodes, none more than 6 cm in greatest dimension, without extranodal extension

    N2c   Metastasis in bilateral or contralateral lymph nodes, none more than 6 cm in greatest dimension, without extranodal extension

N3a   Metastasis in a lymph node more than 6 cm in greatest dimension without extranodal extension

N3b   Metastasis in a single or multiple lymph nodes with clinical extranodal extension*

Note

* The presence of skin involvement or soft tissue invasion with deep fixation/tethering to underlying muscle or adjacent structures or clinical signs of nerve involvement is classified as clinical extranodal extension.

M – Distant Metastasis

M0   No distant metastasis

M1   Distant metastasis

pTNM Pathological Classification

The pT categories correspond to the clinical T categories. For pM see page 8.

pN – Regional Lymph Nodes

Histological examination of a selective neck dissection specimen will ordinarily include 10 or more lymph nodes. Histological examination of a radical or modified radical neck dissection specimen will ordinarily include 15 or more lymph nodes.

pNX   Regional lymph nodes cannot be assessed

pN0   No regional lymph node metastasis

pN1   Metastasis in a single ipsilateral lymph node, 3 cm or less in greatest dimension without extranodal extension

pN2   Metastasis described as:

    pN2a   Metastasis in a single ipsilateral lymph node, less than 3 cm in greatest dimension with extranodal extension or, more than 3 cm but not more than 6 cm in greatest dimension without extranodal extension

    pN2b   Metastasis in multiple ipsilateral lymph nodes, none more than 6 cm in greatest dimension, without extranodal extension

    pN2c   Metastasis in bilateral or contralateral lymph nodes, none more than 6 cm in greatest dimension, without extranodal extension

pN3a   Metastasis in a lymph node more than 6 cm in greatest dimension without extranodal extension

pN3b   Metastasis in a lymph node more than 3 cm in greatest dimension with extranodal extension or multiple ipsilateral, or any contralateral or bilateral node(s) with extranodal extension

Stage

Stage 0	Tis	N0	M0
Stage I	T1	N0	M0
Stage II	T2	N0	M0
Stage III	T3	N0	M0
	T1,T2,T3	N1	M0
Stage IVA	T1,T2,T3	N2, N3	M0
	T4	Any N	M0
Stage IVB	Any T	Any N	M1

Carcinoma of Skin of the Eyelid (ICD-O C44.1)

Rules of Classification

There should be histological confirmation of the disease and division of cases by histological type – for example, basal cell, squamous cell, sebaceous carcinoma. Melanoma of the eyelid is classified with skin tumours, see page 142.

The following are procedures for assessing T, N, and M categories:

T *categories*	Physical examination
N *categories*	Physical examination
M *categories*	Physical examination and imaging

Regional Lymph Nodes

The regional lymph nodes are the preauricular, submandibular, and cervical lymph nodes.

TNM Clinical Classification

T – Primary Tumour

T0 No evidence of primary tumour
Tis Carcinoma in situ

T1 Tumour 10 mm or less in greatest dimension
    T1a Not invading the tarsal plate or eyelid margin
    T1b Invades tarsal plate or eyelid margin
    T1c Involves full thickness of eyelid
T2 Tumour >10 mm, but 20 mm or less in greatest dimension
    T2a Not invading the tarsal plate or eyelid margin
    T2b Invades the tarsal plate or eyelid margin
    T2c Involves full thickness of eyelid
T3 Tumour > 20 mm, but more than 30 mm in greatest dimension
    T3a Not invading the tarsal plate or eyelid margin
    T3b Invades tarsal plate or eyelid margin
    T3c Involves full thickness of eyelid

Skin

T4   Any eyelid tumour that invades adjacent ocular, or orbital, or facial structures

  T4a   Tumour invades ocular or intraorbital structures

  T4b   Tumour invades (or erodes through) the bony walls of orbit or extends to paranasal sinuses or invades the lacrimal sac/nasolacrimal duct or brain

N – Regional Lymph Nodes

NX   Regional lymph nodes cannot be assessed

N0   No evidence of lymph node involvement

N1   Metastasis in a single ipsilateral regional lymph node, 3 cm or less in greatest dimension

N2   Metastasis in a single ipsilateral lymph node more than 3 cm in greatest dimension or in bilateral or contralateral lymph nodes

M – Distant Metastasis

M0   No distant metastasis

M1   Distant metastasis

pTNM Pathological Classification

The pT and pN categories correspond to the T and N categories. For pM see page 8.

Stage

Stage			
Stage 0	Tis	N0	M0
Stage IA	T1	N0	M0
Stage IB	T2a	N0	M0
Stage IIA	T2b, T2c, T3	N0	M0
Stage IIB	T4	N0	M0
Stage IIIA	Any T	N1	M0
Stage IIIB	Any T	N2	M0
Stage IV	Any T	Any N	M1

Prognostic Factor Grid – Eyelid

Prognostic factors for survival for eyelid cancers

Prognostic factors	Tumour related	Host related	Environment related
Essential	Location (worse prognosis if tumour involves the orbit or sinus)	Immunosuppression Periauricular and/or cervical lymph node involvement Systemic metastatic disease at presentation	
Additional	BCC: nodular better than morpheaform type Sebaceous tumours have a worse prognosis than BCC or SCC		
New and promising	Improvements in local control have been associated with less systemic recurrence		

Source: UICC Manual of Clinical Oncology, Ninth Edition. Edited by Brian O'Sullivan, James D. Brierley, Anil K. D'Cruz, Martin F. Fey, Raphael Pollock, Jan B. Vermorken and Shao Hui Huang. © 2015 UICC. Published 2015 by John Wiley & Sons, Ltd.

Malignant Melanoma of Skin
(ICD-O-3 C44, C51.0, C60.9, C63.2)

Rules for Classification

There should be histological confirmation of the disease.

The following are the procedures for assessing N and M categories:

N *categories*   Physical examination and imaging
M *categories*   Physical examination and imaging

Regional Lymph Nodes

The regional lymph nodes are those appropriate to the site of the primary tumour. See page 8.

TNM Clinical Classification

T – Primary Tumour

The extent of the tumour is classified after excision, see pT, page 143.

N – Regional Lymph Nodes

NX   Regional lymph nodes cannot be assessed
N0   No regional lymph node metastasis
N1   Metastasis in one regional lymph node or intralymphatic regional metastasis *without* nodal metastases
    N1a   Only microscopic metastasis (clinically occult)
    N1b   Macroscopic metastasis (clinically apparent)
    N1c   Satellite or in-transit metastasis *without* regional nodal metastasis
N2   Metastasis in two or three regional lymph nodes or intralymphatic regional metastasis *with* lymph node metastases
    N2a   Only microscopic nodal metastasis
    N2b   Macroscopic nodal metastasis
    N2c   Satellite or in-transit metastasis *with* only one regional nodal metastasis
N3   Metastasis in four or more regional lymph nodes, or matted metastatic regional lymph nodes, or satellite(s) or in-transit metastasis *with* metastasis in two or more regional lymph node(s)

N3a Only microscopic nodal metastasis

N3b Macroscopic nodal metastasis

N3c Satellite(s) or in-transit metastasis with two or more regional nodal metastasis

Note

Satellites are tumour nests or nodules (macro- or microscopic) within 2 cm of the primary tumour. In-transit metastasis involves skin or subcutaneous tissue more than 2 cm from the primary tumour but not beyond the regional lymph nodes.

M – Distant Metastasis

M0 No distant metastasis

M1 Distant metastasis*

M1a Skin, subcutaneous tissue or lymph node(s) beyond the regional lymph nodes

M1b Lung

M1c Other non-central nervous system sites

M1d Central nervous system

Notes

* Suffixes for M category:

(0) lactic dehydrogenase (LDH) – not elevated

(1) LDH – elevated

so that M1a(1) is metastasis in skin, subcutaneous tissue, or lymph node(s) beyond the regional lymph nodes with elevated LDH.

No suffix is used if LDH is not recorded or unspecified.

pTNM Pathological Classification

pT – Primary Tumour

pTX Primary tumour cannot be assessed*

pT0 No evidence of primary tumour

pTis Melanoma in situ (Clark level I) (atypical melanocytic hyperplasia, severe melanocytic dysplasia, not an invasive malignant lesion)

Note

* pTX includes shave biopsies and regressed melanomas.

pT1 Tumour 1 mm or less in thickness

pT1a 0.8 mm or less in thickness without ulceration

pT1b 0.8 mm in thickness with ulceration or more than 0.8 mm but no more than 1mm in thickness, with or without ulceration

Skin

pT2 Tumour more than 1 mm but not more than 2 mm in thickness
    pT2a   without ulceration
    pT2b   with ulceration
pT3 Tumour more than 2 mm but not more than 4 mm in thickness
    pT3a   without ulceration
    pT3b   with ulceration
pT4 Tumour more than 4 mm in thickness
    pT4a   without ulceration
    pT4b   with ulceration

pN – Regional Lymph Nodes

The pN categories correspond to the N categories.

pN0   Histological examination of a regional lymphadenectomy specimen will ordinarily include 6 or more lymph nodes. If the lymph nodes are negative, but the number ordinarily examined is not met, classify as pN0. Classification based solely on sentinel node biopsy without subsequent axillary lymph node dissection is designated (sn) for sentinel node, e.g., (p)N1(sn). (See Introduction, page 7.)

pM – Distant Metastasis

For pM see page 8.

Clinical Stage

Stage 0	pTis	N0	M0
Stage IA	pT1a	N0	M0
Stage IB	pT1b	N0	M0
	pT2a	N0	M0
Stage IIA	pT2b	N0	M0
	pT3a	N0	M0
Stage IIB	pT3b	N0	M0
	pT4a	N0	M0
Stage IIC	pT4b	N0	M0
Stage III	Any pT	N1, N2, N3	M0
Stage IV	Any pT	Any N	M1

Pathological Stage*

Stage			
Stage 0	pTis	N0	M0
Stage I	pT1	N0	M0
Stage IA	pT1a	N0	M0
	pT1b	N0	M0
Stage IB	pT2a	N0	M0
Stage IIA	pT2b	N0	M0
	pT3a	N0	M0
Stage IIB	pT3b	N0	M0
	pT4a	N0	M0
Stage IIC	pT4b	N0	M0
Stage III	Any pT	N1, N2, N3	M0
Stage IIIA	pT1a, T1b, T2a	N1a, N2a	M0
Stage IIIB	pT1a, T1b, T2a	N1b, N1c, N2b	M0
	pT2b–T3a	N1, N2a, N2b,	M0
Stage IIIC	pT1a, T1b, T2a, T2b, T3a	N2c, N3	M0
	pT3b, T4a	N1, N2, N3	M0
	pT4b	N1, N2	
Stage IIID	pT4b	N3	M0
Stage IV	Any pT	Any N	M1

*Note. If lymph node(s) are identified with no apparent primary the stage is as below

Stage IIIB	T0	N1b, N1c	M0
Stage IIIC	T0	N2b, N2c, N3b, N3c	M0

Skin

Prognostic Factors Grid – Malignant Melanoma

Prognostic factors for melanoma

Prognostic factors	Tumour related	Host related	Environment related
Essential	Tumour thickness Mitotic rate Ulceration Extent of metastatic disease	Lymphocyte infiltrate Regression	Medications, especially immuno-suppressives
Additional	Lymphovascular Perineural	Site of primary, Family history Personal medical history, especially immunodeficiency Gender (female more favourable) Age (younger age more favourable)	Sun exposure History Tanning bed use
New and promising	Molecular: mutational, gene expression, proteomics, miRNA	Immunogenetics Other characteristics of host immune response	

Source: UICC Manual of Clinical Oncology, Ninth Edition. Edited by Brian O'Sullivan, James D. Brierley, Anil K. D'Cruz, Martin F. Fey, Raphael Pollock, Jan B. Vermorken and Shao Hui Huang. © 2015 UICC. Published 2015 by John Wiley & Sons, Ltd.

Merkel Cell Carcinoma of Skin
(ICD-O-3 C44.0-9, C63.2)

Rules for Classification

The classification applies only to Merkel cell carcinomas. There should be histological confirmation of the disease.

The following are the procedures for assessing T, N, and M categories:

T *categories*   Physical examination
N *categories*   Physical examination and imaging
M *categories*   Physical examination and imaging

Regional Lymph Nodes

The regional lymph nodes are those appropriate to the site of the primary tumour. See page 8.

TNM Clinical Classification

T – Primary Tumour

TX   Primary tumour cannot be assessed
T0   No evidence of primary tumour
Tis Carcinoma in situ

T1   Tumour 2 cm or less in greatest dimension
T2   Tumour more than 2 cm but not more than 5 cm in greatest dimension
T3   Tumour more than 5 cm in greatest dimension
T4   Tumour invades deep extradermal structures, i.e., cartilage, skeletal muscle, fascia or bone

N – Regional Lymph Nodes

NX   Regional lymph nodes cannot be assessed
N0   No regional lymph node metastasis
N1   Regional lymph node metastasis
N2   In-transit metastasis without lymph node metastasis
N3   In-transit metastasis with lymph node metastasis

Note

In-transit metastasis: a discontinuous tumour distinct from the primary lesion and located between the primary lesion and the draining regional lymph nodes or distal to the primary lesion.

M – Distant Metastasis

M0   No distant metastasis
M1   Distant metastasis
      M1a   Skin, subcutaneous tissues or non-regional lymph node(s)
      M1b   Lung
      M1c   Other site(s)

pTNM Pathological Classification

The pT category corresponds to the T category. For pM see page 8.

pN0   Histological examination of a regional lymphadenectomy specimen will ordinarily include 6 or more lymph nodes. If the lymph nodes are negative, but the number ordinarily examined is not met, classify as pN0.

pNX   Regional lymph nodes cannot be assessed
pN0   No regional lymph node metastasis
pN1   Regional lymph node metastasis
      pN1a(sn)   Microscopic metastasis detected on sentinel node biopsy
      pN1a   Microscopic metastasis detected on node dissection
      pN1b   Macroscopic metastasis (clinically apparent)
pN2   In-transit metastasis *without* lymph node metastasis
pN3   In-transit metastasis *with* lymph node metastasis

Note

In-transit metastasis: a discontinuous tumour distinct from the primary lesion and located between the primary lesion and the draining regional lymph nodes or distal to the primary lesion.

Clinical Stage

Stage 0	Tis	N0	M0
Stage I	T1	N0	M0
Stage IIA	T2, T3	N0	M0
Stage IIB	T4	N0	M0
Stage III	Any T	N1, N2, N3	M0
Stage IV	Any T	Any N	M1

Pathological Stage

Stage 0	Tis	N0	M0
Stage I	T1	N0	M0
Stage IIA	T2, T3	N0	M0
Stage IIB	T4	N0	M0
Stage IIIA	T0	N1b	M0
	T1, T2, T3, T4	N1a, N1a(sn)	M0
Stage IIIB	Any T	N1b, N2, N3	M0
Stage IV	Any T	Any N	M1

Skin

Breast Tumours
(ICD-O-3 C50)

Introductory Notes

The site is described under the following headings:

- Rules for classification with the procedures for assessing T, N, and M categories; additional methods may be used when they enhance the accuracy of appraisal before treatment
- Anatomical subsites
- Definition of the regional lymph nodes
- TNM clinical classification
- pTNM pathological classification
- G histopathological grading
- Stage
- Prognostic grid

Rules for Classification

The classification applies only to carcinomas and concerns the male as well as the female breast. There should be histological confirmation of the disease. The anatomical subsite of origin should be recorded but is not considered in classification.

In the case of multiple simultaneous primary tumours in one breast, the tumour with the highest T category should be used for classification. Simultaneous bilateral breast cancers should be classified independently to permit division of cases by histological type.

The following are the procedures for assessing T, N, and M categories:

T categories	Physical examination and imaging, e.g., mammography
N categories	Physical examination and imaging
M categories	Physical examination and imaging

TNM Classification of Malignant Tumours, Eighth Edition. Edited by James D. Brierley, Mary K. Gospodarowicz and Christian Wittekind.
© 2017 UICC. Published 2017 by John Wiley & Sons, Ltd.

Breast

Anatomical Subsites

1. Nipple (C50.0)
2. Central portion (C50.1)
3. Upper-inner quadrant (C50.2)
4. Lower-inner quadrant (C50.3)
5. Upper-outer quadrant (C50.4)
6. Lower-outer quadrant (C50.5)
7. Axillary tail (C50.6)

Regional Lymph Nodes

The regional lymph nodes are:
1. *Axillary* (ipsilateral): interpectoral (Rotter) nodes and lymph nodes along the axillary vein and its tributaries, which may be divided into the following levels:
   a) *Level I* (low-axilla): lymph nodes lateral to the lateral border of pectoralis minor muscle
   b) *Level II* (mid-axilla): lymph nodes between the medial and lateral borders of the pectoralis minor muscle and the interpectoral (Rotter) lymph nodes
   c) *Level III* (apical axilla): apical lymph nodes and those medial to the medial margin of the pectoralis minor muscle, excluding those designated as subclavicular or infraclavicular
2. *Infraclavicular (subclavicular)* (ipsilateral)
3. *Internal mammary* (ipsilateral): lymph nodes in the intercostal spaces along the edge of the sternum in the endothoracic fascia
4. *Supraclavicular* (ipsilateral)

Note
Intramammary lymph nodes are coded as axillary lymph nodes level I. Any other lymph node metastasis is coded as a distant metastasis (M1), including cervical or contralateral internal mammary lymph nodes.

TNM Clinical Classification

T – Primary Tumour

TX	Primary tumour cannot be assessed
T0	No evidence of primary tumour
Tis	Carcinoma in situ
Tis (DCIS)	Ductal carcinoma in situ

Tis (LCIS)	Lobular carcinoma in situ[a]
Tis (Paget)	Paget disease of the nipple not associated with invasive carcinoma and/or carcinoma in situ (DCIS and/or LCIS) in the underlying breast parenchyma. Carcinomas in the breast parenchyma associated with Paget disease are categorized based on the size and characteristics of the parenchymal disease, although the presence of Paget disease should still be noted.

T1	Tumour 2 cm or less in greatest dimension	
	T1mi	Microinvasion 0.1 cm or less in greatest dimension[b]
	T1a	More than 0.1 cm but not more than 0.5 cm in greatest dimension
	T1b	More than 0.5 cm but not more than 1 cm in greatest dimension
	T1c	More than 1 cm but not more than 2 cm in greatest dimension
T2	Tumour more than 2 cm but not more than 5 cm in greatest dimension	
T3	Tumour more than 5 cm in greatest dimension	
T4	Tumour of any size with direct extension to chest wall and/or to skin (ulceration or skin nodules)[c]	
	T4a	Extension to chest wall (does not include pectoralis muscle invasion only)
	T4b	Ulceration, ipsilateral satellite skin nodules, or skin oedema (including peau d'orange)
	T4c	Both 4a and 4b
T4d	Inflammatory carcinoma[d]	

Notes

[a] The AJCC exclude Tis (LCIS).

[b] Microinvasion is the extension of cancer cells beyond the basement membrane into the adjacent tissues with no focus more than 0.1 cm in greatest dimension. When there are multiple foci of microinvasion, the size of only the largest focus is used to classify the microinvasion. (Do not use the sum of all individual foci.) The presence of multiple foci of microinvasion should be noted, as it is with multiple larger invasive carcinomas.

[c] Invasion of the dermis alone does not qualify as T4. Chest wall includes ribs, intercostal muscles, and serratus anterior muscle but not pectoral muscle.

[d] Inflammatory carcinoma of the breast is characterized by diffuse, brawny induration of the skin with an erysipeloid edge, usually with no underlying mass. If the skin biopsy is negative and there is no localized measurable primary cancer, the T category is pTX when pathologically staging a clinical inflammatory carcinoma (T4d). Dimpling of the skin, nipple retraction, or other skin changes, except those in T4b and T4d, may occur in T1, T2, or T3 without affecting the classification.

Breast

N – Regional Lymph Nodes

NX   Regional lymph nodes cannot be assessed (e.g., previously removed)

N0   No regional lymph node metastasis

N1   Metastasis in movable ipsilateral level I, II axillary lymph node(s)

N2   Metastasis in ipsilateral level I, II axillary lymph node(s) that are clinically fixed or matted; or in clinically detected* ipsilateral internal mammary lymph node(s) in the *absence* of clinically evident axillary lymph node metastasis

     N2a   Metastasis in axillary lymph node(s) fixed to one another (matted) or to other structures

     N2b   Metastasis only in clinically detected* internal mammary lymph node(s) and in the *absence* of clinically detected axillary lymph node metastasis

N3   Metastasis in ipsilateral infraclavicular (level III axillary) lymph node(s) with or without level I, II axillary lymph node involvement; or in clinically detected* ipsilateral internal mammary lymph node(s) with clinically evident level I, II axillary lymph node metastasis; or metastasis in ipsilateral supraclavicular lymph node(s) with or without axillary or internal mammary lymph node involvement

     N3a   Metastasis in infraclavicular lymph node(s)

     N3b   Metastasis in internal mammary and axillary lymph nodes

     N3c   Metastasis in supraclavicular lymph node(s)

Notes

* Clinically detected is defined as detected by clinical examination or by imaging studies (excluding lymphoscintigraphy) and having characteristics highly suspicious for malignancy or a presumed pathological macrometastasis based on fine needle aspiration biopsy with cytological examination. Confirmation of clinically detected metastatic disease by fine needle aspiration without excision biopsy is designated with a (f) suffix, e.g. cN3a(f).

Excisional biopsy of a lymph node or biopsy of a sentinel node, in the absence of assignment of a pT, is classified as a clinical N, e.g., cN1. Pathological classification (pN) is used for excision or sentinel lymph node biopsy only in conjunction with a pathological T assignment.

M – Distant Metastasis

M0   No distant metastasis

M1   Distant metastasis

pTNM Pathological Classification

pT – Primary Tumour

The pathological classification requires the examination of the primary carcinoma with no gross tumour at the margins of resection. A case can be classified pT if there is only microscopic tumour in a margin.

The pT categories correspond to the T categories.

Note

When classifying pT the tumour size is a measurement of the invasive component. If there is a large in situ component (e.g., 4 cm) and a small invasive component (e.g., 0.5 cm), the tumour is coded pT1a.

pN – Regional Lymph Nodes

The pathological classification requires the resection and examination of at least the low axillary lymph nodes (level I) (see page 152). Such a resection will ordinarily include 6 or more lymph nodes. If the lymph nodes are negative, but the number ordinarily examined is not met, classify as pN0.

pNX Regional lymph nodes cannot be assessed (e g , previously removed, or not removed for pathological study)

pN0 No regional lymph node metastasis*

Note

* Isolated tumour cell clusters (ITC) are single tumour cells or small clusters of cells not more than 0.2 mm in greatest extent that can be detected by routine H and E stains or immunohistochemistry. An additional criterion has been proposed to include a cluster of fewer than 200 cells in a single histological cross section. Nodes containing only ITCs are excluded from the total positive node count for purposes of N classification and should be included in the total number of nodes evaluated. (See Introduction, page 7.)

pN1 Micrometastases; or metastases in 1 to 3 axillary ipsilateral lymph nodes; and/or in internal mammary nodes with metastases detected by sentinel lymph node biopsy but not clinically detected*

    pN1mi Micrometastases (larger than 0.2 mm and/or more than 200 cells, but none larger than 2.0 mm)

    pN1a Metastasis in 1–3 axillary lymph node(s), including at least one larger than 2 mm in greatest dimension

    pN1b Internal mammary lymph nodes

    pN1c Metastasis in 1–3 axillary lymph nodes and internal mammary lymph nodes.

pN2   Metastasis in 4–9 ipsilateral axillary lymph nodes, or in clinically detected* ipsilateral internal mammary lymph node(s) in the absence of axillary lymph node metastasis

    pN2a   Metastasis in 4–9 axillary lymph nodes, including at least one that is larger than 2 mm

    pN2b   Metastasis in clinically detected internal mammary lymph node(s), in the *absence* of axillary lymph node metastasis

pN3

    pN3a   Metastasis in 10 or more ipsilateral axillary lymph nodes (at least one larger than 2 mm) or metastasis in infraclavicular lymph nodes

    pN3b   Metastasis in clinically detected* internal ipsilateral mammary lymph node(s) in the *presence* of positive axillary lymph node(s); or metastasis in more than 3 axillary lymph nodes *and* in internal mammary lymph nodes with microscopic or macroscopic metastasis detected by sentinel lymph node biopsy but not clinically detected

    pN3c   Metastasis in ipsilateral supraclavicular lymph node(s)

Post-treatment ypN:

- Post-treatment yp 'N' should be evaluated as for clinical (pretreatment) 'N' methods (see Section N – Regional Lymph Nodes). The modifier 'sn' is used only if a sentinel node evaluation was performed after treatment. If no subscript is attached, it is assumed the axillary nodal evaluation was by axillary node dissection.
- The X classification will be used (ypNX) if no yp post-treatment SN or axillary dissection was performed
- N categories are the same as those used for pN.

Notes

* *Clinically detected* is defined as detected by imaging studies (excluding lymphoscintigraphy) or by clinical examination and having characteristics highly suspicious for malignancy or a presumed pathological macrometastasis based on fine needle aspiration biopsy with cytological examination.

Not clinically detected is defined as not detected by imaging studies (excluding lymphoscintigraphy) or not detected by clinical examination.

pM – Distant Metastasis

For pM see page 8.

G Histopathological Grading

For histopathological grading of invasive carcinoma the Nottingham Histological Score is recommended.[1]

Stage[a]

Stage 0	Tis	N0	M0
Stage IA	T1[b]	N0	M0
Stage IB	T0, T1	N1mi	M0
Stage IIA	T0, T1	N1	M0
	T2	N0	M0
Stage IIB	T2	N1	M0
	T3	N0	M0
Stage IIIA	T0, T1, T2	N2	M0
	T3	N1, N2	M0
Stage IIIB	T4	N0, N1, N2	M0
Stage IIIC	Any T	N3	M0
Stage IV	Any T	Any N	M1

Notes

[a] The AJCC also publish a prognostic group for breast tumours.

[b] T1 includes T1mi.

Prognostic Factors Grid – Breast

Prognostic factors for breast cancer

Prognostic factors	Tumour related	Host related	Environment related
Essential	ER HER2 receptor Histological grade Number and percentage of involved nodes Tumour size Presence of lymphatic or vascular invasion (LVI+) Surgical resection margin status	Age Menopausal status	Prior radiation involving the chest or mediastinum (e.g. for Hodgkin disease)
Additional	Progesterone receptor Tumour profiling UPA, PAI-1	BRCA1 or 2 mutation Obesity	Use of postmenopausal hormone replacement therapy
New and promising	Ki-67	Level of activity or exercise Single nucleotide polymorphisms (SNPs) associated with drug metabolism or action	

Source: UICC Manual of Clinical Oncology, Ninth Edition. Edited by Brian O'Sullivan, James D. Brierley, Anil K. D'Cruz, Martin F. Fey, Raphael Pollock, Jan B. Vermorken and Shao Hui Huang. © 2015 UICC. Published 2015 by John Wiley & Sons, Ltd.

Reference

1 Elston CW, Ellis IO. Pathological prognostic factors in breast cancer. I. The value of histological grade in breast cancer: experience from a large study with long-term follow-up. *Histopathology* 1991; 19: 403–410.

Gynaecological Tumours

Introductory Notes

The following sites are included:
- Vulva
- Vagina
- Cervix uteri
- Corpus uteri
  - Endometrium
  - Uterine sarcomas
- Ovary, fallopian tube and primary peritoneal carcinoma
- Gestational trophoblastic tumours

Cervix uteri and corpus uteri were among the first sites to be classified by the TNM system. Originally, carcinoma of the cervix uteri was staged following the rules suggested by the Radiological Sub-Commission of the Cancer Commission of the Health Organization of The League of Nations. These rules were then adopted, with minor modifications, by the newly formed Fédération Internationale de Gynécologie et d'Obstétrique (FIGO). Finally, UICC brought them into the TNM in order to correspond to the FIGO stages. FIGO, UICC, and AJCC work in close collaboration in the revision process. The classification of tumours of ovary and fallopian tube has been revised in line with the recent FIGO update.[1]

Each site is described under the following headings:
- Rules for classification with the procedures for assessing T, N, and M categories; additional methods may be used when they enhance the accuracy of appraisal before treatment
- Anatomical subsites where appropriate
- Definition of the regional lymph nodes
- TNM clinical classification
- pTNM pathological classification
- Stage
- Prognostic grid

Gynaecological

TNM Classification of Malignant Tumours, Eighth Edition. Edited by James D. Brierley, Mary K. Gospodarowicz and Christian Wittekind.
© 2017 UICC. Published 2017 by John Wiley & Sons, Ltd.

Histopathological Grading

The definitions of the G categories apply to all carcinomas. These are:

G – Histopathological Grading

GX   Grade of differentiation cannot be assessed
G1   Well differentiated
G2   Moderately differentiated
G3   Poorly differentiated or undifferentiated

Reference

1 Prat J, FIGO Committee on Gynecologic Oncology. Staging classification for cancer of the ovary, fallopian tube, and peritoneum. *Int J Gynecol Obstet* 2014; 124: 1–5.

Vulva
(ICD-O-3 C51)

The definitions of the T, N, and M categories correspond to the FIGO stages.

Rules for Classification

The classification applies only to primary carcinomas of the vulva. There should be histological confirmation of the disease.

A carcinoma of the vulva that has extended to the vagina is classified as carcinoma of the vulva.

The following are the procedures for assessing T, N, and M categories:

T *categories*   Physical examination, endoscopy, and imaging
N *categories*   Physical examination and imaging
M *categories*   Physical examination and imaging

The FIGO stages are based on surgical staging. (TNM stages are based on clinical and/or pathological classification.)

Regional Lymph Nodes

The regional lymph nodes are the inguinofemoral (groin) nodes.

TNM Clinical Classification

T – Primary tumour

TX   Primary tumour cannot be assessed
T0   No evidence of primary tumour
Tis   Carcinoma in situ (preinvasive carcinoma), intraepithelial neoplasia grade III (VIN III)

T1   Tumour confined to vulva or vulva and perineum
  T1a   Tumour 2 cm or less in greatest dimension and with stromal invasion no greater than 1.0 mm[a]
  T1b   Tumour greater than 2 cm and or with stromal invasion greater than 1 mm[a]
T2   Tumour invades any of the following structures: lower third urethra, lower third vagina, anus

T3[b] Tumour invades any of the following perineal structures: upper 2/3 urethra, upper 2/3 vagina, bladder mucosa, rectal mucosa; or fixed to pelvic bone

Notes

[a] The depth of invasion is defined as the measurement of the tumour from the epithelial–stromal junction of the adjacent most superficial dermal papilla to the deepest point of invasion.

[b] T3 is not used by FIGO.

N – Regional Lymph Nodes

NX Regional lymph nodes cannot be assessed
N0 No regional lymph node metastasis
N1 Regional lymph node metastasis with the following features:
    N1a One or two lymph node metastasis each less than 5 mm
    N1b One lymph node metastases 5 mm or greater
N2 Regional lymph node metastasis with the following features:
    N2a Three or more lymph node metastases each less than 5 mm
    N2b Two or more lymph node metastases 5 mm or greater
    N2c Lymph node metastasis with extracapsular spread
N3 Fixed or ulcerated regional lymph node metastasis

M – Distant Metastasis

M0 No distant metastasis
M1 Distant metastasis (including pelvic lymph node metastasis)

pTNM Pathological Classification

The pT and pN categories correspond to the T and N categories. For pM see page 8.

pN0 Histological examination of an inguinofemoral lymphadenectomy specimen will ordinarily include 6 or more lymph nodes. If the lymph nodes are negative, but the number ordinarily examined is not met, classify as pN0.

Stage

Stage 0	Tis	N0	M0
Stage I	T1	N0	M0
Stage IA	T1a	N0	M0

Stage IB	T1b	N0	M0
Stage II	T2	N0	M0
Stage IIIA	T1, T2	N1a, N1b	M0
Stage IIIB	T1, T2	N2a, N2b	M0
Stage IIIC	T1, T2	N2c	M0
Stage IVA	T1, T2	N3	M0
	T3	Any N	M0
Stage IVB	Any T	Any N	M1

Prognostic Factors Grid – Vulva

Prognostic risk factors for cancer of the vulva

Prognostic factors	Tumour related	Host related	Environment related
Essential	Lymph node metastases: • Number • Size • Extracapsular tumour growth		Experience of treating centre/concentration of care for vulvar cancer patients in tertiary referral centres
Additional	FIGO stage Depth of invasion Diameter of primary tumour Histological type	Age Smoking Adjacent dermatosis (LS, VIN) Immune status	Surgical margins
New and promising	EGFR status p53 over-expression P16INK4a level Microvessel density	HPV status Pretreatment haemoglobin level	

Source: UICC Manual of Clinical Oncology, Ninth Edition. Edited by Brian O'Sullivan, James D. Brierley, Anil K. D'Cruz, Martin F. Fey, Raphael Pollock, Jan B. Vermorken and Shao Hui Huang. © 2015 UICC. Published 2015 by John Wiley & Sons, Ltd.

Gynaecological

Vagina
(ICD-O-3 C52)

The definitions of the T and M categories correspond to the FIGO stages. Both systems are included for comparison.

Rules for Classification

The classification applies to primary carcinomas only. Tumours present in the vagina as secondary growths from either genital or extragenital sites are excluded. A tumour that has extended to the portio and reached the external os (orifice of uterus) is classified as carcinoma of the cervix. A vaginal carcinoma occurring 5 years after successful treatment (complete response) of a carcinoma of the cervix uteri is considered a primary vaginal carcinoma. A tumour involving the vulva is classified as carcinoma of the vulva. There should be histological confirmation of the disease.

The following are the procedures for assessing T, N, and M categories:

T categories	Physical examination, endoscopy, and imaging
N categories	Physical examination and imaging
M categories	Physical examination and imaging

The FIGO stages are based on surgical staging. (TNM stages are based on clinical and/or pathological classification.)

Regional Lymph Nodes

Upper two-thirds of vagina: the pelvic nodes including obturator, internal iliac (hypogastric), external iliac, and pelvic nodes, NOS.
Lower third of vagina: the inguinal and femoral nodes.

TNM Clinical Classification

T – Primary Tumour

TNM Categories	FIGO Stages	Definition
TX		Primary tumour cannot be assessed
T0		No evidence of primary tumour
Tis		Carcinoma in situ (preinvasive carcinoma)
T1	I	Tumour confined to vagina

TNM Categories	FIGO Stages	Definition
T2	II	Tumour invades paravaginal tissues (paracolpium)
T3	III	Tumour extends to pelvic wall
T4	IVA	Tumour invades mucosa of bladder or rectum, or extends beyond the true pelvis*
M1	IVB	Distant metastasis

Note

* The presence of bullous oedema is not sufficient evidence to classify a tumour as T4.

N – Regional Lymph Nodes

NX   Regional lymph nodes cannot be assessed
N0   No regional lymph node metastasis
N1   Regional lymph node metastasis

M – Distant Metastasis

M0   No distant metastasis
M1   Distant metastasis

TNM Pathological Classification

The pT and pN categories correspond to the T and N categories. For pM see page 8.

pN0   Histological examination of an inguinal lymphadenectomy speci men will ordinarily include 6 or more lymph nodes; a pelvic lymphadenectomy specimen will ordinarily include 10 or more lymph nodes. If the lymph nodes are negative, but the number ordinarily examined is not met, classify as pN0.

Stage

Stage			
Stage 0	Tis	N0	M0
Stage I	T1	N0	M0
Stage II	T2	N0	M0
Stage III	T3	N0	M0
	T1, T2, T3	N1	M0
Stage IVA	T4	Any N	M0
Stage IVB	Any T	Any N	M1

Gynaecological

Cervix Uteri
(ICD-O C53)

The definitions of the T and M categories correspond to the FIGO stages. Both systems are included for comparison.

Rules for Classification

The classification applies only to carcinomas. There should be histological confirmation of the disease.

The following are the procedures for assessing T, N, and M categories:

T *categories*	Clinical examination and imaging*
N *categories*	Clinical examination and imaging
M *categories*	Clinical examination and imaging

Note

* The use of diagnostic imaging techniques to assess the size of the primary tumour is encouraged but is not mandatory. Other investigations, e.g., examination under anaesthesia, cystoscopy, sigmoidoscopy, intravenous pyelography, are optional and no longer mandatory.

The FIGO stages are based on clinical staging. For some Stage I subdivisions (IA–IB1) are mainly pathological, including the histological examination of the cervix. (TNM stages are based on clinical and/or pathological classification.)

Anatomical Subsites

1. Endocervix (C53.0)
2. Exocervix (C53.1)

Regional Lymph Nodes

The regional lymph nodes are the paracervical, parametrial, hypogastric (internal iliac, obturator), common and external iliac, presacral, and lateral sacral nodes. Para-aortic nodes are not regional.

TNM Clinical Classification

T – Primary Tumour

TNM Categories	FIGO Stages	Definition
TX		Primary tumour cannot be assessed
T0		No evidence of primary tumour
Tis		Carcinoma in situ (preinvasive carcinoma)
T1	I	Tumour confined to the cervix[a]
T1a[b,c]	IA	Invasive carcinoma diagnosed only by microscopy. Stromal invasion with a maximal depth of 5.0 mm measured from the base of the epithelium and a horizontal spread of 7.0 mm or less[d]
T1a1	IA1	Measured stromal invasion 3.0 mm or less in depth and 7.0 mm or less in horizontal spread
T1a2	IA2	Measured stromal invasion more than 3.0 mm and not more than 5.0 mm with a horizontal spread of 7.0 mm or less
T1b	IB	Clinically visible lesion confined to the cervix or microscopic lesion greater than T1a/IA2
T1b1	IB1	Clinically visible lesion 4.0 cm or less in greatest dimension
T1b2	IB2	Clinically visible lesion more than 4.0 cm in greatest dimension
T2	II	Tumour invades beyond uterus but not to pelvic wall or to lower third of vagina
T2a	IIA	Tumour without parametrial invasion
T2a1	IIA1	Clinically visible lesion 4.0 cm or less in greatest dimension

(Continued)

Gynaecological

(Continued)

TNM Categories	FIGO Stages	Definition
T2a2	IIA2	Clinically visible lesion more than 4.0 cm in greatest dimension
T2b	IIB	Tumour with parametrial invasion
T3	III	Tumour, involves lower third of vagina, or extends to pelvic wall, or causes hydronephrosis or non-functioning kidney
T3a	IIIA	Tumour involves lower third of vagina
T3b	IIIB	Tumour extends to pelvic wall, or causes hydronephrosis or non-functioning kidney
T4	IVA	Tumour invades mucosa of the bladder or rectum, or extends beyond true pelvis[e]

Notes

[a] Extension to corpus uteri should be disregarded.

[b] The depth of invasion should be taken from the base of the epithelium, either surface or glandular, from which it originates. The depth of invasion is defined as the measurement of the tumour from the epithelial–stromal junction of the adjacent most superficial papillae to the deepest point of invasion.

Vascular space involvement, venous or lymphatic, does not affect classification.

[c] All macroscopically visible lesions even with superficial invasion are T1b/IB.

[d] Vascular space involvement, venous or lymphatic, does not affect classification.

[e] Bullous oedema is not sufficient to classify a tumour as T4.

N – Regional lymph nodes*

NX   Regional lymph nodes cannot be assessed
N0   No regional lymph node metastasis
N1   Regional lymph node metastasis

Note

* No FIGO equivalent.

M – Distant Metastasis

M0   No distant metastasis
M1   Distant metastasis (includes inguinal lymph nodes and intraperitoneal disease). It excludes metastasis to vagina, pelvic serosa, and adnexa

pTNM Pathological Classification

The pT and pN categories correspond to the T and N categories. For pM see page 8.

pN0   Histological examination of a pelvic lymphadenectomy specimen will ordinarily include 10 or more lymph nodes. If the lymph nodes are negative, but the number ordinarily examined is not met, classify as pN0.

Stage

Stage			
Stage 0	Tis	N0	M0
Stage I	T1	N0	M0
Stage IA	T1a	N0	M0
Stage IA1	T1a1	N0	M0
Stage IA2	T1a2	N0	M0
Stage IB	T1b	N0	M0
Stage IB1	T1b1	N0	M0
Stage IB2	T1b2	N0	M0
Stage II	T2	N0	M0
Stage IIA	T2a	N0	M0
Stage IIA1	T2a1	N0	M0
Stage IIA2	T2a2	N0	M0
Stage IIB	T2b	N0	M0
Stage III	T3	N0	M0
Stage IIIA	T3a	N0	M0
Stage IIIB	T3b	Any N	M0
	T1, T2, T3	N1	M0
Stage IVA	T4	Any N	M0
Stage IVB	Any T	Any N	M1

Prognostic Factors Grid – Cervix Uteri

Prognostic risk factors in cervical cancer

Prognostic factors	Tumour related	Host related	Environment related
Essential	Unilateral vs bilateral disease Parametrial invasion Invasion to side wall Size of tumour Lymph node invasion Positive surgical margins	Immunosuppression (i.e. HIV infection) Performance status Morbid obesity	Quality of and availability of anticancer therapies Expertise of healthcare personnel Multidisciplinary teams
Additional	Lymphovascular space invasion Histological type	Anaemia during treatment	Ability to manage co-morbid conditions
New and promising	Tumour hypoxia VEGF, mEGFR, HIF-1α, COX-2 PAI-1 expression SCC-Ag and hsCRP for early detection of recurrence	Serum MyoDI hypermethylation Persistence of HPV infection following treatment	Adequate laboratory facilities to measure tumour markers

Source: UICC Manual of Clinical Oncology, Ninth Edition. Edited by Brian O'Sullivan, James D. Brierley, Anil K. D'Cruz, Martin F. Fey, Raphael Pollock, Jan B. Vermorken and Shao Hui Huang. © 2015 UICC. Published 2015 by John Wiley & Sons, Ltd.

Uterus – Endometrium
(ICD-O-3 C54.1, C55)

The definitions of the T, N, and M categories correspond to the FIGO stages. Both systems are included for comparison.

Rules for Classification

The classification applies to endometrial carcinomas and carcinosarcomas (malignant mixed mesodermal tumours). There should be histological verification with subdivision by histological type and grading of the carcinomas. The diagnosis should be based on examination of specimens taken by endometrial biopsy.

The following are the procedures for assessing T, N, and M categories:

T categories	Physical examination and imaging including urography and cystoscopy
N categories	Physical examination and imaging including urography
M categories	Physical examination and imaging.

The FIGO stages are based on surgical staging. (TNM stages are based on clinical and/or pathological classification.)

Anatomical Subsites

1. Isthmus uteri (C54.0)
2. Fundus uteri (C54.3)
3. Endometrium (C54.1)

Regional Lymph Nodes

The regional lymph nodes are the pelvic (hypogastric [obturator, internal iliac], common and external iliac, parametrial, and sacral) and the para-aortic nodes.

Gynaecological

TNM Clinical Classification

T – Primary Tumour

TNM Categories		FIGO Stages	
TX			Primary tumour cannot be assessed
T0			No evidence of primary tumour
T1		I[a]	Tumour confined to the corpus uteri[a]
	T1a	IA[a]	Tumour limited to endometrium or invading less than half of myometrium
	T1b	IB	Tumour invades one half or more of myometrium
T2		II	Tumour invades cervical stroma, but does not extend beyond the uterus
T3		III	Local and/or regional spread as specified here:
	T3a	IIIA	Tumour invades the serosa of the corpus uteri or adnexae (direct extension or metastasis)
	T3b	IIIB	Vaginal or parametrial involvement (direct extension or metastasis)
N1,N2		IIIC	Metastasis to pelvic or para-aortic lymph nodes[b]
	N1	IIIC1	Metastasis to pelvic lymph nodes
	N2	IIIC2	Metastastis to para-aortic lymph nodes with or without metastasis to pelvic lymph nodes
T4[c]		IV	Tumour invades bladder/bowel mucosa

Notes

[a] Endocervical glandular involvement only should be considered as stage I.

[b] Positive cytology has to be reported separately without changing the stage.

[c] The presence of bullous oedema is not sufficient evidence to classify as T4.

N – Regional Lymph Nodes

NX Regional lymph nodes cannot be assessed
N0 No regional lymph node metastasis
N1 Regional lymph node metastasis to pelvic lymph nodes
N2 Regional lymph node metastasis to para-aortic lymph nodes with or without metastasis to pelvic lymph nodes

M – Distant Metastasis

M0 No distant metastasis
M1 Distant metastasis (excluding metastasis to vagina, pelvic serosa, or adnexa, including metastasis to inguinal lymph nodes, intra-abdominal lymph nodes other than para-aortic or pelvic nodes)

pTNM Pathological Classification

The pT and pN categories correspond to the T and N categories. For pM see page 8.

pN0 Histological examination of a pelvic lymphadenectomy specimen will ordinarily include 10 or more lymph nodes. If the lymph nodes are negative, but the number ordinarily examined is not met, classify as pN0.

G Histopathological Grading

For histopathological grading use G1, G2, or G3. For details see Creasman et al. 2006.[1]

Stage

Stage 0	Tis	N0	M0
Stage IA	T1a	N0	M0
Stage IB	T1b	N0	M0
Stage II	T2	N0	M0
Stage IIIA	T3a	N0	M0
Stage IIIB	T3b	N0	M0
Stage III	T1, T2, T3	N1, N2	M0

Stage IIIC1	T1, T2, T3	N1	M0
Stage IIIC2	T1, T2, T3	N2	M0
Stage IVA	T4	Any N	M0
Stage IVB	Any T	Any N	M1

Prognostic Grid – Endometrium

Prognostic factors for endometrial carcinoma

Prognostic factors	Tumour related	Host related	Environment related
Essential	Depth of myometrial invasion Grade of differentiation Tumour cell type Lymphovascular space invasion		Postsurgical treatment
Additional	Metastasis to lymph nodes Site of distant metastasis	Age Performance status Race Co-morbidities	Extent of resection Postsurgical treatment
New and promising	Molecular profile		

Source: UICC Manual of Clinical Oncology, Ninth Edition. Edited by Brian O'Sullivan, James D. Brierley, Anil K. D'Cruz, Martin F. Fey, Raphael Pollock, Jan B. Vermorken and Shao Hui Huang. © 2015 UICC. Published 2015 by John Wiley & Sons, Ltd.

Reference

1 Creasman WT, Odicino F, Maisoneuve P, Quinn MA, Beller U, Benedet JL, Heintz APM, Ngan HYS, Pecorelli S. FIGO Annual Report on the results of treatment in gynaecological cancer. Vol. 26. Carcinoma of the corpus uteri. *Int J Gynecol Obstet* 2006; 95 (Suppl. 1): 105–143.

Uterine Sarcomas
(Leiomyosarcoma, Endometrial Stromal Sarcoma, Adenosarcoma) (ICD-O-3 53, 54)

The definitions of the T, N, and M categories correspond to the FIGO stages. Both systems are included for comparison.[1,2]

Rules for Classification

The classification applies to sarcomas except for carcinosarcoma, which is classified as carcinoma of the endometrium. There should be histological confirmation and division of cases by histological type.

The following are the procedures for assessing T, N, and M categories:

T *categories*   Physical examination and imaging
N *categories*   Physical examination and imaging
M *categories*   Physical examination and imaging

The FIGO stages are based on surgical staging. (TNM stages are based on clinical and/or pathological classification.)

Anatomical Subsites

1. Cervix uteri (C53)
2. Isthmus uteri (C54.0)
3. Fundus uteri (C54.3)

Histological Types of Tumours

Leiomyosarcoma	8890/3
Endometrial stromal sarcoma	8930/3
Adenosarcoma	8933/3

Regional Lymph Nodes

The regional lymph nodes are the pelvic (hypogastric [obturator, internal iliac], common and external iliac, parametrial, and sacral) and the para-aortic nodes.

Gynaecological

TNM Clinical Classification

Leiomyosarcoma, Endometrial stromal sarcoma

T – Primary tumour

TNM categories		FIGO Stage	Definition
T1		I	Tumour limited to the uterus
	T1a	IA	Tumour 5 cm or less in greatest dimension
	T1b	IB	Tumour more than 5 cm
T2		II	Tumour extends beyond the uterus, within the pelvis
	T2a	IIA	Tumour involves adnexa
	T2b	IIB	Tumour involves other pelvic tissues
T3		III	Tumour infiltrates abdominal tissues
	T3a	IIIA	One site
	T3b	IIIB	More than one site
N1		IIIC	Metastasis to regional lymph nodes
T4		IVA	Tumour invades bladder or rectum
M1		IVB	Distant metastasis

Note
Simultaneous tumours of the uterine corpus and ovary/pelvis in association with ovarian/pelvic endometriosis should be classified as independent primary tumours.

Adenosarcoma

T – Primary tumour

TNM categories		FIGO Stage	Definition
T1		I	Tumour limited to the uterus
	T1a	IA	Tumour limited to the endometrium/endocervix
	T1b	IB	Tumour invades to less than half of the myometrium

(Continued)

TNM categories		FIGO Stage	Definition
	T1c	IC	Tumour invades more than half of the myometrium
T2		II	Tumour extends beyond the uterus, within the pelvis
	T2a	IIA	Tumour involves adnexa
	T2b	IIB	Tumour involves other pelvic tissues
T3		III	Tumour involves abdominal tissues
	T3a	IIIA	One site
	T3b	IIIB	More than one site
N1		IIIC	Metastasis to regional lymph nodes
T4		IVA	Tumour invades bladder or rectum
M1		IVB	Distant metastasis

Note

Simultaneous tumours of the uterine corpus and ovary/pelvis in association with ovarian/pelvic endometriosis should be classified as independent primary tumours.

N – Regional Lymph Nodes

NX   Regional lymph nodes cannot be assessed
N0   No regional lymph node metastasis
N1   Regional lymph node metastasis

M – Distant Metastasis

M0   No distant metastasis
M1   Distant metastasis (excluding adnexa, pelvic and abdominal tissues)

pTNM Pathological Classification

The pT and pN categories correspond to the T and N categories. For pM see page 8.

Stage – Uterine Sarcomas

Stage I	T1	N0	M0
Stage IA	T1a	N0	M0
Stage IB	T1b	N0	M0
Stage IC*	T1c	N0	M0
Stage II	T2	N0	M0
Stage IIA	T2a	N0	M0
Stage IIB	T2b	N0	M0
Stage IIIA	T3a	N0	M0
Stage IIIB	T3b	N0	M0
Stage IIIC	T1, T2, T3	N1	M0
Stage IVA	T4	Any N	M0
Stage IVB	Any T	Any N	M1

Note

* Stage IC does not apply for leiomyosarcoma and endometrial stromal sarcoma.

References

1 Prat J. FIGO staging for uterine sarcomas. *Int J Gynaecol Obstet* 2009; 104: 177–178.
2 FIGO Committee on Gynecologic Oncology Report. FIGO staging for uterine sarcomas. *Int J Gynaecol Obstet* 2009; 104: 179.

Ovarian, Fallopian Tube, and Primary Peritoneal Carcinoma
(ICD-O-3 C56; ICD-O-3 C57)

The definitions of the T, N, and M categories correspond to the FIGO stages. Both systems are included for comparison.

Rules for Classification

The classification applies to malignant ovarian neoplasms of both epithelial and stromal origin including those of borderline malignancy or of low malignant potential[1] corresponding to 'common epithelial tumours' of the earlier terminology.

The classification also applies to carcinoma of the fallopian tubes and to carcinomas of the peritoneum (Müllerian origin).

There should be histological confirmation of the disease and division of cases by histological type.

The following are the procedures for assessing T, N, and M categories:

T categories	Clinical examination, imaging, surgical exploration (laparoscopy/laparotomy)
N categories	Clinical examination, imaging, surgical exploration (laparoscopy/laparotomy)
M categories	Clinical examination, imaging, surgical exploration (laparoscopy/laparotomy)

The FIGO stages are based on surgical staging. (TNM stages are based on clinical and/or pathological classification.)

Regional Lymph Nodes

The regional lymph nodes are the hypogastric (obturator), common iliac, external iliac, lateral sacral, para-aortic, retroperitoneal, and inguinal nodes.

Gynaecological

TNM Clinical Classification

T – Primary Tumour

TNM categories	FIGO Stage	Definition
TX		Primary tumour cannot be assessed
T0		No evidence of primary tumour
T1	I	Tumour limited to the ovaries (one or both) or fallopian tube(s)
T1a	IA	Tumour limited to one ovary; capsule intact, no tumour on ovarian surface or fallopian tube surface; no malignant cells in ascites or peritoneal washings
T1b	IB	Tumour limited to both ovaries or fallopian tubes; capsule intact, no tumour on ovarian or fallopian tube surface; no malignant cells in ascites or peritoneal washings
T1c	IC	Tumour limited to one or both ovaries or fallopian tubes with any of the following:
T1c1		Surgical spill
T1c2		Capsule ruptured before surgery or tumour on ovarian or fallopian tube surface
T1c3		Malignant cells in ascites or peritoneal washings
T2	II	Tumour involves one or both ovaries or fallopian tubes with pelvic extension (below the pelvic brim) or primary peritoneal cancer
T2a	IIA	Extension and/or implants on uterus and/or fallopian tube(s) and or ovary(ies)
T2b	IIB	Extension to other pelvic tissues, including bowel within the pelvis
T3 and/or N1	III[a]	Tumour involves one or both ovaries or fallopian tubes or primary peritoneal carcinoma with cytologically or histologically confirmed spread to the peritoneum outside the pelvis and/or metastasis to the retroperitoneal lymph nodes

(Continued)

TNM categories		FIGO Stage	Definition
N1			Retroperitoneal lymph node metastasis only
	N1a	IIIA1i	Lymph node metastasis not more than 10 mm in greatest dimension
	N1b	IIIA1ii	Lymph node metastasis more than 10 mm in greatest dimension
T3a any N		IIIA2	Microscopic extrapelvic (above the pelvic brim) peritoneal involvement with or without retroperitoneal lymph node, including bowel involvement
T3b any N		IIIB	Macroscopic peritoneal metastasis beyond pelvic brim 2 cm, or less in greatest dimension, including bowel involvement outside the pelvis with or without retroperitoneal nodes
T3c any N		IIIC	Peritoneal metastasis beyond pelvic brim more than 2 cm in greatest dimension and/or retroperitoneal lymph node metastasis (includes extension of tumour to capsule of liver and spleen without parenchymal involvement of either organ)
M1		IV	Distant metastasis (excludes peritoneal metastasis)
	M1a	IVA	Pleural effusion with positive cytology
	M1b[b]	IVB	Parenchymal metastasis and metastasis to extra-abdominal organs (including inguinal lymph nodes and lymph nodes outside the abdominal cavity)

Notes

[a] Liver capsule metastasis is T3/stage III.

[b] Liver parenchymal metastasis M1/stage IV.

Gynaecological

N – Regional Lymph Nodes

NX Regional lymph nodes cannot be assessed
N0 No regional lymph node metastasis
N1 Regional lymph node metastasis

N1	IIIA1	Retroperitoneal lymph node metastasis only
N1a	IIIA1i	Lymph node metastasis no more than 10 mm in greatest dimension
N1b	IIIA1ii	Lymph node metastasis more than 10 mm in greatest dimension

M – Distant Metastasis

M0 No distant metastasis
M1 Distant metastasis

pTNM Pathological Classification

The pT and pN categories correspond to the T and N categories. For pM see page 8.

pN0 Histological examination of a pelvic lymphadenectomy specimen will ordinarily include 10 or more lymph nodes. If the lymph nodes are negative, but the number ordinarily examined is not met, classify as pN0.

Stage

Stage I	T1	N0	M0
Stage IA	T1a	N0	M0
Stage IB	T1b	N0	M0
Stage IC	T1c	N0	M0
Stage II	T2	N0	M0
Stage IIA	T2a	N0	M0
Stage IIB	T2b	N0	M0
Stage IIC	T2c	N0	M0
Stage IIIA1	T1/2	N1	M0
Stage IIIA2	T3a	N0, N1	M0
Stage IIIB	T3b	N0, N1	M0
Stage IIIC	T3c	N0, N1	M0
Stage IV	Any T	Any N	M1
Stage IVA	Any T	Any N	M1a
Stage IVB	Any T	Any N	M1b

Prognostic Factors Grid – Tumours of the Ovary, Fallopian Tube and Peritoneal Carcinoma

Prognostic risk factor for epithelial ovarian cancer

Prognostic factors	Tumour related	Host related	Environment related
Essential	Histological type Grade Surgical stage Residual disease	Age Co-morbidities Performance status	Maximum diameter of residual disease after optimal debulking
Additional	Nodal involvement Site of metastasis DNA ploidy CA125	BRCA 1 Genetic predisposition	Type of chemotherapy CA125 fall Ultra-radical surgery
New and promising	Molecular profile Cellular proliferative activity Tumour angiogenesis markers p53 expression Expression of human kallikrein (hK) genes, particularly hKs 6-10-11		Interval debulking surgery (IDS) Neoadjuvant chemotherapy

Source: UICC Manual of Clinical Oncology, Ninth Edition. Edited by Brian O'Sullivan, James D. Brierley, Anil K. D'Cruz, Martin F. Fey, Raphael Pollock, Jan B. Vermorken and Shao Hui Huang. © 2015 UICC. Published 2015 by John Wiley & Sons, Ltd.

Reference

1 Tavassoli FA, Devilee P (eds). WHO *Classification of Tumours. Pathology and Genetics. Tumours of the Breast and Female Genital Organs*. Lyon, France: IACR Press, 2003.

Gynaecological

Gestational Trophoblastic Neoplasms (ICD-O-3 C58)

The following classification for gestational trophoblastic tumours is based on that of FIGO adopted in 1992 and updated in 2002.[1] The definitions of T and M categories correspond to the FIGO stages. Both systems are included for comparison. In contrast to other sites, an N (regional lymph node) classification does not apply to these tumours. A prognostic scoring index, which is based on factors other than the anatomic extent of the disease, is used to assign cases to high-risk and low-risk categories, and these categories are used in stage grouping.

Rules for Classification

The classification applies to choriocarcinoma (9100/3), invasive hydatidiform mole (9100/1), and placental site trophoblastic tumour (9104/1). Placental site tumours should be reported separately. Histological confirmation is not required if the human chorionic gonadotropin (βhCG) level is abnormally elevated. History of prior chemotherapy for this disease should be noted.

The following are the procedures for assessing T and M categories:

T *categories:*	Clinical examination, imaging and endoscopy, and serum/urine βhCG level
M *categories:*	Clinical examination, imaging, and assessment of serum/urine βhCG level
Risk *categories:*	Age, type of antecedent pregnancy, interval months from index pregnancy, pretreatment **serum/urine** βhCG, diameter of largest tumour, site of metastasis, number of metastases, and previous failed chemotherapy are integrated to provide a prognostic score that divides cases into low and high-risk categories.

TM Clinical Classification

T – Primary Tumour

TM Categories	FIGO Stages[a]	Definition
TX		Primary tumour cannot be assessed
T0		No evidence of primary tumour
T1	I	Tumour confined to uterus
T2[b]	II	Tumour extends to other genital structures: vagina, ovary, broad ligament, fallopian tube by metastasis or direct extension
M1a	III	Metastasis to lung(s)
M1b[c]	IV	Other distant metastasis

Notes

[a] Stages I to IV are subdivided into A and B according to the prognostic score.

[b] Genital metastasis (vagina, ovary, broad ligament, fallopian tube) is classified T2.

[c] Any involvement of non-genital structures, whether by direct invasion or metastasis is described using the M classification.

pTM Pathological Classification

The pT categories correspond to the T categories. For pM see page 8.

Stage

Stage I	T1	M0
Stage II	T2	M0
Stage III	Any T	M1a
Stage IV	Any T	M1b

Prognostic Score

Prognostic Factor	0	1	2	4
Age	<40	≥40		
Antecedent pregnancy	H. mole	Abortion	Term pregnancy	
Months from index pregnancy	<4	4–6	7–12	>12
Pretreatment serum hCG (IU/ml)	<10^3	10^3–<10^4	10^4–<10^5	>10^5
Largest tumour size including uterus	<3 cm	3–5 cm	>5 cm	
Sites of metastasis	Lung	Spleen, kidney	Gastrointestinal tract	Liver, brain
Number of metastasis		1–4	5–8	>8
Previous failed chemotherapy			Single drug	Two or more drugs

Risk categories:

Total prognostic score 6 or less = low risk

Total score 7 or more = high risk

Prognostic Group

Record stage and prognostic score separated by a colon, i.e., **II: 4 or IV: 9**

Reference

1 Ngan HYS, Bender H, Benedet JL, Jones H, Montrucolli GC, Pecorelli S; FIGO Committee on Gynecologic Oncology. Gestational trophoblastic neoplasia. *Int J Gynecol Obstet* 2002; 77: 285–287.

Urological Tumours

Introductory Notes

The following sites are included:
- Penis
- Prostate
- Testis
- Kidney
- Renal pelvis and ureter
- Urinary bladder
- Urethra

Each site is described under the following headings:
- Rules for classification with the procedures for assessing T, N, and M categories; additional methods may be used when they enhance the accuracy of appraisal before treatment
- Anatomical sites and subsites where appropriate
- Definition of the regional lymph nodes
- Distant metastasis
- TNM clinical classification
- pTNM pathological classification
- G Histopathological grading where applicable
- Stage
- Prognostic factors grid

TNM Classification of Malignant Tumours, Eighth Edition. Edited by James D. Brierley, Mary K. Gospodarowicz and Christian Wittekind.
© 2017 UICC. Published 2017 by John Wiley & Sons, Ltd.

Penis
(ICD-O-3 C60)

Rules for Classification

The classification applies only to carcinomas. There should be histological confirmation of the disease.

The following are the procedures for assessing T, N, and M categories:

T *categories*   Physical examination and endoscopy
N *categories*   Physical examination and imaging
M *categories*   Physical examination and imaging

Anatomical Subsites

1. Prepuce (C60.0)
2. Glans penis (C60.1)
3. Body of penis (C60.2)

Regional Lymph Nodes

The regional lymph nodes are the superficial and deep inguinal and the pelvic nodes.

TNM Clinical Classification

T – Primary Tumour

TX   Primary tumour cannot be assessed
T0   No evidence of primary tumour
Tis   Carcinoma in situ
Ta   Non-invasive verrucous carcinoma*

T1   Tumour invades subepithelial connective tissue
    T1a   Tumour invades subepithelial connective tissue without lymphovascular invasion and is not poorly differentiated
    T1b   Tumour invades subepithelial connective tissue with lymphovascular invasion or is poorly differentiated
T2   Tumour invades corpus spongiosum with or without invasion of the urethra
T3   Tumour invades corpus cavernosum with or without invasion of the urethra
T4   Tumour invades other adjacent structures

Note

* Verrucous carcinoma not associated with destructive invasion.

N – Regional Lymph Nodes

NX   Regional lymph nodes cannot be assessed

N0   No palpable or visibly enlarged inguinal lymph nodes

N1   Palpable mobile unilateral inguinal lymph node

N2   Palpable mobile multiple or bilateral inguinal lymph nodes

N3   Fixed inguinal nodal mass or pelvic lymphadenopathy unilateral or bilateral

M – Distant Metastasis

M0   No distant metastasis

M1   Distant metastasis

pTNM Pathological Classification

The pT categories correspond to the T categories. The pN categories are based upon biopsy, or surgical excision. For pM see page 8.

pNX   Regional lymph nodes cannot be assessed

pN0   No regional lymph node metastasis

pN1   Metastasis in one or two inguinal lymph nodes

pN2   Metastasis in more than two unilateral inguinal nodes or bilateral inguinal lymph nodes

pN3   Metastasis in pelvic lymph node(s), unilateral or bilateral or extranodal extension of regional lymph node metastasis

Stage

Stage 0	Tis	N0	M0
	Ta	N0	M0
Stage I	T1a	N0	M0
Stage IIA	T1b, T2	N0	M0
Stage IIB	T3	N0	M0
Stage IIIA	T1, T2, T3	N1	M0
Stage IIIB	T1, T2, T3	N2	M0
Stage IV	T4	Any N	M0
	Any T	N3	M0
	Any T	Any N	M1

Prognostic Factors Grid – Penis

Prognostic factors for survival for squamous cell carcinoma

Prognostic factor	Tumour related	Host related	Environment related
Essential	Differentiation Lymphovascular space invasion Invasion of the corpora	History of genital condylomas Lichen sclerosis PUVA	Poor hygiene
Additional	HPV/p16 (presence may confer better prognosis)	Smoking HIV/immune suppression	
New and promising	p53 (predicts for lymph node metastases) EGFR		

Source: UICC Manual of Clinical Oncology, Ninth Edition. Edited by Brian O'Sullivan, James D. Brierley, Anil K. D'Cruz, Martin F. Fey, Raphael Pollock, Jan B. Vermorken and Shao Hui Huang. © 2015 UICC. Published 2015 by John Wiley & Sons, Ltd.

Prostate
(ICD-O-3 C61.9)

Rules for Classification

The classification applies only to adenocarcinomas. Transitional cell carcinoma of the prostate is classified as a urethral tumour (see page 208). There should be histological confirmation of the disease.

The following are the procedures for assessing T, N, and M categories:

T *categories*   Physical examination, imaging, endoscopy, biopsy, and biochemical tests

N *categories*   Physical examination and imaging

M *categories*   Physical examination, imaging, skeletal studies, and biochemical tests

Regional Lymph Nodes

The regional lymph nodes are the nodes of the true pelvis, which essentially are the pelvic nodes below the bifurcation of the common iliac arteries. Laterality does not affect the N classification.

TNM Clinical Classification

T – Primary Tumour

TX   Primary tumour cannot be assessed
T0   No evidence of primary tumour

T1   Clinically inapparent tumour that is not palpable
    T1a   Tumour incidental histological finding in 5% or less of tissue resected
    T1b   Tumour incidental histological finding in more than 5% of tissue resected
    T1c   Tumour identified by needle biopsy (e.g., because of elevated PSA)
T2   Tumour that is palpable and confined within prostate
    T2a   Tumour involves one half of one lobe or less
    T2b   Tumour involves more than half of one lobe, but not both lobes
    T2c   Tumour involves both lobes

T3   Tumour extends through the prostatic capsule*

    T3a Extracapsular extension (unilateral or bilateral) including microscopic bladder neck involvement

    T3b Tumour invades seminal vesicle(s)

T4   Tumour is fixed or invades adjacent structures other than seminal vesicles: external sphincter, rectum, levator muscles, and/or pelvic wall

Note

* Invasion into the prostatic apex or into (but not beyond) the prostatic capsule is not classified as T3, but as T2.

N – Regional Lymph Nodes

NX   Regional lymph nodes cannot be assessed

N0   No regional lymph node metastasis

N1   Regional lymph node metastasis

Note

Metastasis no larger than 0.2 cm can be designated pNmi. (See Introduction, pN, page 7.)

M – Distant Metastasis*

M0   No distant metastasis

M1   Distant metastasis

    M1a Non-regional lymph node(s)

    M1b Bone(s)

    M1c Other site(s)

Note

* When more than one site of metastasis is present, the most advanced category is used. (p)M1c is the most advanced category.

pTNM Pathological Classification

The pT and pN categories correspond to the T and N categories. For pM see page 8.

However, there is no pT1 category because there is insufficient tissue to assess the highest pT category or subcategories of pT2.

G Histopathological Grade Group[1,2]

GX   Grade cannot be assessed

Grade Group	Gleason Score	Gleason Pattern
1	≤6	≤3 + 3
2	7	3 + 4
3	7	4 + 3
4	8	4 + 4
5	9–10	4 + 5, 5 + 4, 5 + 5

Stage*

Stage I	T1, T2a	N0	M0
Stage II	T2b, T2c	N0	M0
Stage III	T3, T4	N0	M0
Stage IV	Any T	N1	M0
	Any T	Any N	M1

Note

* The AJCC also publish a prognostic group for prostate tumours.

Prognostic Factors Grid – Prostate

Prognostic factors for prostate cancer

Prognostic factor	Tumour related	Host related	Environment related
Essential	Gleason sum score Grade group TNM stage PSA level	Co-morbidity Age Performance status	
Additional	Alkaline phosphatase (if bone metastases) % involvement of cores on biopsy and number of positive cores		

Source: UICC Manual of Clinical Oncology, Ninth Edition. Edited by Brian O'Sullivan, James D. Brierley, Anil K. D'Cruz, Martin F. Fey, Raphael Pollock, Jan B. Vermorken and Shao Hui Huang. © 2015 UICC. Published 2015 by John Wiley & Sons, Ltd.

References

1 Epstein JI, Egevad L, Amin MB, et al. The 2014 International Society of Urological Pathology (ISUP) Consensus Conference on Gleason Grading of Prostatic Carcinoma: Definition of Grading Patterns and Proposal for a New Grading System. *Am J Surg Pathol* 2016; 40: 244–252.

2 Humphrey PA, Egevard L, Netto GL, et al. Acinar adenocarcinoma. In: *WHO Classification of Tumours of the Urinary System and Male Genital Organs*. Moch H, et al., eds. Lyon, France: IACR, 2016.

Testis
(ICD-O-3 C62)

Rules for Classification

The classification applies only to germ cell tumours of the testis. There should be histological confirmation of the disease and division of cases by histological type. Histopathological grading is not applicable.

The presence of elevated serum tumour markers, including alpha-fetoprotein (AFP), human chorionic gonadotropin (hCG), and lactate dehydrogenase (LDH), is frequent in this disease. Staging is based on the determination of the anatomic extent of disease and assessment of serum tumour markers.

The following are the procedures for assessing N, M, and S categories:

N *categories*   Physical examination and imaging
M *categories*   Physical examination, imaging, and biochemical tests
S *categories*   Serum tumour markers

Stages are subdivided based on the presence and degree of elevation of serum tumour markers. Serum tumour markers are obtained immediately after orchiectomy and, if elevated, should be performed serially after orchiectomy according to the normal decay for AFP (half-life 7 days) and hCG (half-life 3 days) to assess for serum tumour marker elevation. The S classification is based on the nadir value of hCG and AFP after orchiectomy. The serum level of LDH (but not its half-life levels) has prognostic value in patients with metastatic disease and is included for staging.

Regional Lymph Nodes

The regional lymph nodes are the abdominal para-aortic (periaortic), preaortic, interaortocaval, precaval, paracaval, retrocaval, and retroaortic nodes. Nodes along the spermatic vein should be considered regional. Laterality does not affect the N classification. The intrapelvic nodes and the inguinal nodes are considered regional after scrotal or inguinal surgery.

TNM Clinical Classification

T – Primary tumour

Except for pTis and pT4, where radical orchiectomy is not always necessary for classification purposes, the extent of the primary tumour is classified after radical orchiectomy; see pT. In other circumstances, TX is used if no radical orchiectomy has been performed.

N – Regional Lymph Nodes

NX Regional lymph nodes cannot be assessed
N0 No regional lymph node metastasis
N1 Metastasis with a lymph node mass 2 cm or less in greatest dimension or multiple lymph nodes, none more than 2 cm in greatest dimension
N2 Metastasis with a lymph node mass more than 2 cm but not more than 5 cm in greatest dimension, or multiple lymph nodes, any one mass more than 2 cm but not more than 5 cm in greatest dimension
N3 Metastasis with a lymph node mass more than 5 cm in greatest dimension

M – Distant Metastasis

M0 No distant metastasis
M1 Distant metastasis
    M1a Non-regional lymph node(s) or lung metastasis
    M1b Distant metastasis other than non-regional lymph nodes and lung

pTNM Pathological Classification

pT – Primary Tumour

pTX Primary tumour cannot be assessed (see T – Primary Tumour)
pT0 No evidence of primary tumour (e.g., histological scar in testis)
pTis Intratubular germ cell neoplasia (carcinoma in situ)

pT1 Tumour limited to testis and epididymis without vascular/lymphatic invasion; tumour may invade tunica albuginea but not tunica vaginalis*
pT2 Tumour limited to testis and epididymis with vascular/lymphatic invasion, or tumour extending through tunica albuginea with involvement of tunica vaginalis
pT3 Tumour invades spermatic cord with or without vascular/lymphatic invasion
pT4 Tumour invades scrotum with or without vascular/lymphatic invasion

Note

* AJCC subdivides T1 by T1a and T1b depending on size no greater than 3 cm or greater than 3 cm in greatest dimension.

pN – Regional Lymph Nodes

pNX   Regional lymph nodes cannot be assessed

pN0   No regional lymph node metastasis

pN1   Metastasis with a lymph node mass 2 cm or less in greatest dimension and 5 or fewer positive nodes, none more than 2 cm in greatest dimension

pN2   Metastasis with a lymph node mass more than 2 cm but not more than 5 cm in greatest dimension; or more than 5 nodes positive, none more than 5 cm; or evidence of extranodal extension of tumour

pN3   Metastasis with a lymph node mass more than 5 cm in greatest dimension

pM – Distant Metastasis

For pM see page 8.

S – Serum Tumour Markers

SX   Serum marker studies not available or not performed

S0   Serum marker study levels within normal limits

	LDH	hCG (mIU/ml)	AFP (ng/ml)
S1	$<1.5 \times N$	and <5000	and <1000
S2	$1.5–10 \times N$	or 5000–50 000	or 1000–10 000
S3	$>10 \times N$	or $>50 000$	or $>10 000$

Note

N indicates the upper limit of normal for the LDH assay.

Prognostic group

Stage 0	pTis	N0	M0	S0
Stage I	pT1–T4	N0	M0	SX
Stage IA	pT1	N0	M0	S0
Stage IB	pT2–T4	N0	M0	S0

Stage IS	Any pT/TX	N0	M0	S1 – S3
Stage II	Any pT/TX	N1 – N3	M0	SX
Stage IIA	Any pT/TX	N1	M0	S0
	Any pT/TX	N1	M0	S1
Stage IIB	Any pT/TX	N2	M0	S0
	Any pT/TX	N2	M0	S1
Stage II	Any pT/TX	N3	M0	S0
	Any pT/TX	N3	M0	S1
Stage III	Any pT/TX	Any N	M1a	SX
Stage IIIA	Any pT/TX	Any N	M1a	S0
	Any pT/TX	Any N	M1a	S1
Stage IIIB	Any pT/TX	N1–N3	M0	S2
	Any pT/TX	Any N	M1a	S2
Stage IIIC	Any pT/TX	N1–N3	M0	S3
	Any pT/TX	Any N	M1a	S3
	Any pT/TX	Any N	M1b	Any S

Prognostic Factors Grid – Testis

Prognostic factors for testicular cancer

Prognostic factors	Tumour related	Host related	Environment related
Essential	Histological type T category N category M category Tumour markers (AFP, hCG, LDH) Site of metastases		
Additional	Rate of marker decline	Delay in diagnosis	Physician expertise
New and promising	Copy number of i(12p) p53 Ki-67 Apoptotic index		

Source: UICC Manual of Clinical Oncology, Ninth Edition. Edited by Brian O'Sullivan, James D. Brierley, Anil K. D'Cruz, Martin F. Fey, Raphael Pollock, Jan B. Vermorken and Shao Hui Huang. © 2015 UICC. Published 2015 by John Wiley & Sons, Ltd.

Kidney
(ICD-O-3 C64)

Rules for Classification

The classification applies only to renal cell carcinoma. There should be histological confirmation of the disease.

The following are the procedures for assessing T, N, and M categories:

T categories	Physical examination and imaging
N categories	Physical examination and imaging
M categories	Physical examination and imaging

Regional Lymph Nodes

The regional lymph nodes are the hilar, abdominal para-aortic, and para-caval nodes. Laterality does not affect the N categories.

TNM Clinical Classification

T – Primary Tumour

TX   Primary tumour cannot be assessed
T0   No evidence of primary tumour

T1   Tumour 7 cm or less in greatest dimension, limited to the kidney
     T1a   Tumour 4 cm or less
     T1b   Tumour more than 4 cm but not more than 7 cm
T2   Tumour more than 7 cm in greatest dimension, limited to the kidney
     T2a   Tumour more than 7 cm but not more than 10 cm
     T2b   Tumour more than 10 cm, limited to the kidney
T3   Tumour extends into major veins or perinephric tissues but not into the ipsilateral adrenal gland and not beyond Gerota fascia
     T3a   Tumour grossly extends into the renal vein or its segmental (muscle containing) branches, or tumour invades perirenal and/or renal sinus fat (peripelvic) fat but not beyond Gerota fascia
     T3b   Tumour grossly extends into vena cava below diaphragm
     T3c   Tumour grossly extends into vena cava above the diaphragm or invades the wall of the vena cava
T4   Tumour invades beyond Gerota fascia (including contiguous extension into the ipsilateral adrenal gland)

N – Regional Lymph Nodes

NX   Regional lymph nodes cannot be assessed
N0   No regional lymph node metastasis
N1   Metastasis in regional lymph node(s)

M – Distant Metastasis

M0   No distant metastasis
M1   Distant metastasis

pTNM Pathological Classification

The pT and pN categories correspond to the T and N categories. For pM see page 8.

Stage

Stage I	T1	N0	M0
Stage II	T2	N0	M0
Stage III	T3	N0	M0
	T1, T2, T3	N1	M0
Stage IV	T4	Any N	M0
	Any T	Any N	M1

Prognostic Factors Grid – Kidney

Prognostic factors for cancers of the kidney

Prognostic factors	Tumour related	Host related	Environment related
Essential	Stage	Surgical candidacy	
Additional	Histological subtype Fuhrman grade (clear cell RCC only) Histological features of necrosis, sarcomatoid histology Symptom score	Performance status Hereditary diseases	Lymph node dissection Adrenalectomy Metastatectomy Immunotherapy/targeted therapy
Investigational	DNA ploidy Genetic alterations Molecular markers		

Renal Pelvis and Ureter
(ICD-O-3 C65, C66)

Rules for Classification

The classification applies to carcinomas. Papilloma is excluded. There should be histological or cytological confirmation of the disease.

The following are the procedures for assessing T, N, and M categories:

T *categories*   Physical examination, imaging, and endoscopy
N *categories*   Physical examination and imaging
M *categories*   Physical examination and imaging

Anatomical Sites

1. Renal pelvis (C65)
2. Ureter (C66)

Regional Lymph Nodes

The regional lymph nodes are the hilar, abdominal para-aortic, and para-caval nodes and, for ureter, intrapelvic nodes. Laterality does not affect the N classification.

TNM Clinical Classification

T – Primary Tumour

TX   Primary tumour cannot be assessed
T0   No evidence of primary tumour
Ta   Non-invasive papillary carcinoma
Tis   Carcinoma in situ

T1   Tumour invades subepithelial connective tissue
T2   Tumour invades muscularis
T3   (*Renal pelvis*) Tumour invades beyond muscularis into peripelvic fat or renal parenchyma
      (*Ureter*) Tumour invades beyond muscularis into periureteric fat
T4   Tumour invades adjacent organs or through the kidney into perinephric fat

N – Regional Lymph Nodes

NX   Regional lymph nodes cannot be assessed
N0   No regional lymph node metastasis
N1   Metastasis in a single lymph node 2 cm or less in greatest dimension
N2   Metastasis in a single lymph node more than 2 cm, or multiple lymph
     nodes

M – Distant Metastasis

M0   No distant metastasis
M1   Distant metastasis

pTNM Pathological Classification

The pT and pN categories correspond to the T and N categories. For pM
see page 8.

Stage

Stage 0a	Ta	N0	M0
Stage 0is	Tis	N0	M0
Stage I	T1	N0	M0
Stage II	T2	N0	M0
Stage III	T3	N0	M0
Stage IV	T4	N0	M0
	Any T	N1, N2	M0
	Any T	Any N	M1

Urinary Bladder
(ICD-O-3 C67)

Rules for Classification

The classification applies to carcinomas. Papilloma is excluded. There should be histological or cytological confirmation of the disease.

The following are the procedures for assessing T, N, and M categories:

T *categories*   Physical examination, imaging, and endoscopy
N *categories*   Physical examination and imaging
M *categories*   Physical examination and imaging

Regional Lymph Nodes

The regional lymph nodes are the nodes of the true pelvis, which essentially are the pelvic nodes below the bifurcation of the common iliac arteries. Laterality does not affect the N classification.

TNM Clinical Classification

T – Primary Tumour

The suffix (m) should be added to the appropriate T category to indicate multiple tumours. The suffix (is) may be added to any T to indicate presence of associated carcinoma in situ.

TX   Primary tumour cannot be assessed
T0   No evidence of primary tumour
Ta   Non-invasive papillary carcinoma
Tis   Carcinoma in situ: 'flat tumour'

T1   Tumour invades subepithelial connective tissue
T2   Tumour invades muscle
    T2a   Tumour invades superficial muscle (inner half)
    T2b   Tumour invades deep muscle (outer half)
T3   Tumour invades perivesical tissue:
    T3a   microscopically
    T3b   macroscopically (extravesical mass)

T4   Tumour invades any of the following: prostate stroma, seminal vesicles, uterus, vagina, pelvic wall, abdominal wall

    T4a   Tumour invades prostate stroma, seminal vesicles, uterus or vagina

    T4b   Tumour invades pelvic wall or abdominal wall

N – Regional Lymph Nodes

NX   Regional lymph nodes cannot be assessed

N0   No regional lymph node metastasis

N1   Metastasis in a single lymph node in the true pelvis (hypogastric, obturator, external iliac, or presacral)

N2   Metastasis in multiple regional lymph nodes in the true pelvis (hypogastric, obturator, external iliac, or presacral)

N3   Metastasis in a common iliac lymph node(s)

M – Distant Metastasis

M0   No distant metastasis

    M1a   Non-regional lymph nodes

    M1b   Other distant metastasis

pTNM Pathological Classification

The pT and pN categories correspond to the T and N categories. For pM see page 8.

Stage

Stage 0a	Ta	N0	M0
Stage 0is	Tis	N0	M0
Stage I	T1	N0	M0
Stage II	T2a, T2b	N0	M0
Stage IIIA	T3a, T3b, T4a	N0	M0
	T1, T2, T3, T4a	N1	M0
Stage IIIB	T1, T2, T3, T4a	N2, N3	M0
Stage IVA	T4b	N0	M0
	Any T	Any N	M1a
Stage IVB	Any T	Any N	M1b

Prognostic Factors Grid – Bladder

Prognostic factors for progression to invasive disease in superficial bladder cancer (Ta, T1, Tis)

Prognostic factor	Tumour related	Host related	Environment related
Essential	Grade T stage Carcinoma in situ (Cis) Number of lesions Previous recurrences	Age Performance status Other co-morbidities	Extent of transurethral resection (Intravesical chemotherapy reduces recurrence but limited evidence for reducing progression)
Additional	Tumour size Recurrence at 3-month check	Gender Continued tobacco use	
Novel/ promising	p53 NMP22 FGFR3 mutation status COX-2 (especially upper tract) Claudin protein family members DNA methylation status Lymphovascular invasion Extent of invasion (T1 microinvasive or T1 extensive invasive)		

Prognostic factors for metastatic risk and survival in invasive, locally-advanced and/or node positive bladder cancer (T2–4 N0–1)

Prognostic factors	Tumor related	Host related	Environment related
Essential	T category N category	Age Performance status ALP Other co-morbidities	Surgical margin status
Additional	Grade Histological type Lymphovascular invasion Concomitant Cis Tumour size Hydronephrosis	Haemoglobin Response of primary to chemotherapy	Extent of lymph node resection Proportion (density) of involved lymph nodes
Novel/ promising	p53, p63, p21 (for long-term bladder preservation) Rb protein Ki67 EGF receptor HER2 expression E-cadherin Microvessel density Treatment resistance mechanisms (ERCC1, BRCA1 or MMR mutations)	Certain germline singlenucleotide polymorphisms (SNPs)	

With established metastatic disease, visceral metastasis is associated with a poorer prognosis.

Source: UICC Manual of Clinical Oncology, Ninth Edition. Edited by Brian O'Sullivan, James D. Brierley, Anil K. D'Cruz, Martin F. Fey, Raphael Pollock, Jan B. Vermorken and Shao Hui Huang. © 2015 UICC. Published 2015 by John Wiley & Sons, Ltd.

Urethra
(ICD-O-3 C68.0, C61.9)

Rules for Classification

The classification applies to carcinomas of the urethra (ICD-O C68.0) and transitional cell carcinomas of the prostate (ICD-O C61.9) and prostatic urethra. There should be histological or cytological confirmation of the disease.

The following are the procedures for assessing T, N, and M categories:

T *categories*   Physical examination, imaging, and endoscopy
N *categories*   Physical examination and imaging
M *categories*   Physical examination and imaging

Regional Lymph Nodes

The regional lymph nodes are the inguinal and the pelvic nodes. Laterality does not affect the N classification.

TNM Clinical Classification

T – Primary Tumour

TX   Primary tumour cannot be assessed
T0   No evidence of primary tumour

Urethra (male and female)
Ta   Non-invasive papillary, polypoid, or verrucous carcinoma
Tis   Carcinoma in situ

T1   Tumour invades subepithelial connective tissue
T2   Tumour invades any of the following: corpus spongiosum, prostate, periurethral muscle
T3   Tumour invades any of the following: corpus cavernosum, beyond prostatic capsule, anterior vagina, bladder neck (extraprostatic extension)
T4   Tumour invades other adjacent organs (invasion of the bladder)

Urothelial (transitional cell) carcinoma of the prostate
Tis pu   Carcinoma in situ, involvement of prostatic urethra
Tis pd   Carcinoma in situ, involvement of prostatic ducts

T1 Tumour invades subepithelial connective tissue (for tumours involving prostatic urethra only)

T2 Tumour invades any of the following: prostatic stroma, corpus spongiosum, periurethral muscle

T3 Tumour invades any of the following: corpus cavernosum, beyond prostatic capsule, bladder neck (extraprostatic extension)

T4 Tumour invades other adjacent organs (invasion of the bladder or rectum)

N – Regional Lymph Nodes

NX Regional lymph nodes cannot be assessed
N0 No regional lymph node metastasis
N1 Metastasis in a single lymph node
N2 Metastasis in multiple lymph nodes

M – Distant Metastasis

M0 No distant metastasis
M1 Distant metastasis

pTNM Pathological Classification

The pT and pN categories correspond to the T and N categories. For pM see page 8.

Stage

Stage 0a	Ta	N0	M0
Stage 0is	Tis	N0	M0
Stage I	T1	N0	M0
Stage II	T2	N0	M0
Stage III	T1, T2	N1	M0
	T3	N0, N1	M0
Stage IV	T4	N0, N1	M0
	Any T	N2	M0
	Any T	Any N	M1

Adrenal Cortex
(ICD-O-3 C74.0)

Rules for Classification

This classification applies only to carcinomas of the adrenal cortex. It does not apply to tumours of the adrenal medulla or sarcomas.

The following are the procedures for assessing T, N, and M categories:

T categories   Physical examination and imaging
N categories   Physical examination and imaging
M categories   Physical examination and imaging

Regional Lymph Nodes

The regional lymph nodes are the hilar, abdominal para-aortic, and para-caval nodes. Laterality does not affect the N categories.

TNM Clinical Classification

T – Primary Tumour

TX   Primary tumour cannot be assessed
T0   No evidence of primary tumour

T1   Tumour 5 cm or less in greatest dimension, no extra-adrenal invasion
T2   Tumour greater than 5 cm, no extra-adrenal invasion
T3   Tumour of any size with local invasion, but not invading adjacent organs*
T4   Tumour of any size with invasion of adjacent organs*

Note
* Adjacent organs include kidney, diaphragm, great vessels (renal vein or vena cava), pancreas, and liver.

TNM Classification of Malignant Tumours, Eighth Edition. Edited by James D. Brierley, Mary K. Gospodarowicz and Christian Wittekind.
© 2017 UICC. Published 2017 by John Wiley & Sons, Ltd.

N – Regional lymph nodes

NX   Regional lymph nodes cannot be assessed
N0   No regional lymph node metastasis
N1   Metastasis in regional lymph node(s)

M – Distant Metastasis

M0   No distance metastasis
M1   Distant metastasis

pTNM Pathological Classification

The pT and pN categories correspond to the T and N categories. For pM see page 8.

Stage

Stage I	T1	N0	M0
Stage II	T2	N0	M0
Stage III	T1, T2	N1	M0
	T3, T4	N0, N1	M0
Stage IV	Any T	Any N	M1

Prognostic Factors Grid

Prognostic factors for survival in ACC

Prognostic factors	Tumour related	Host related	Environment related
Essential	T, N, M categories Biochemical status: • Improved survival in patients with functional tumours		Resectability
Additional	Response to mitotane	Age	
New and promising	Molecular profile: • Higher tumour grade, described by Ki-67 or mitotic rate is associated with poorer prognosis • Chromosomal aberrations associated with poor survival: gain in chromosomes 6, 7, 12 and 19; and loss in chromosomes 3, 8, 10, 16, 17 and 19 • Increasing degree of aberration is associated with shorter survival		

Source: UICC Manual of Clinical Oncology, Ninth Edition. Edited by Brian O'Sullivan, James D. Brierley, Anil K. D'Cruz, Martin F. Fey, Raphael Pollock, Jan B. Vermorken and Shao Hui Huang. © 2015 UICC. Published 2015 by John Wiley & Sons, Ltd.

Ophthalmic Tumours

Introductory Notes

Tumours of the eye and its adnexa are a disparate group including carcinoma, melanoma, sarcomas, and retinoblastoma. For clinical convenience they are classified in one section.

The following sites are included:

- Eyelid (eyelid tumours are classified with skin tumours)
- Conjunctiva
- Uvea
- Retina
- Orbit
- Lacrimal gland

For histological nomenclature and diagnostic criteria, reference to the WHO histological classification is recommended.[1]

Each tumour type is described under the following headings:

- Rules for classification with the procedures for assessing the T, N, and M categories
- Anatomical sites where appropriate
- Definition of the regional lymph nodes
- TNM clinical classification
- pTNM pathological classification
- Stage where applicable
- Prognostic factors grid

Reference

1 Campbell RJ. *Histological Typing of Tumours of the Eye and its Adnexa*, 2nd edn. Berlin: Springer, 1998.

Ophthalmic

TNM Classification of Malignant Tumours, Eighth Edition. Edited by James D. Brierley, Mary K. Gospodarowicz and Christian Wittekind.
© 2017 UICC. Published 2017 by John Wiley & Sons, Ltd.

Carcinoma of Conjunctiva
(ICD-O-3 C 69.0)

Rules for Classification

There should be histological confirmation of the disease and division of cases by histological type, for example, mucoepidermoid and squamous cell carcinoma.

The following are the procedures for assessing T, N, and M categories:

T *categories*   Physical examination
N *categories*   Physical examination
M *categories*   Physical examination and imaging

Regional Lymph Nodes

The regional lymph nodes are the preauricular, submandibular and cervical lymph nodes.

TNM Clinical Classification

T – Primary Tumour

TX   Primary tumour cannot be assessed
T0   No evidence of primary tumour
Tis   Carcinoma in situ

T1   Tumour 5 mm or less in greatest dimension invades through the conjuctival basement membrane
T2   Tumour more than 5 mm in greatest dimension, invades through the conjuctival basement membrane without invasion of adjacent structures*
T3   Tumour invades adjacent structures*
T4   Tumour invades the orbit or beyond
     T4a   Tumour invades orbital soft tissues, without bone invasion
     T4b   Tumour invades bone
     T4c   Tumour invades adjacent paranasal sinuses
     T4d   Tumour invades brain

Note

* Adjacent structures include: the cornea (3, 6, 9, or 12 clock hours), intraocular compartments, forniceal conjunctiva (lower and/or upper), palpebral conjunctiva (lower and/or upper), tarsal conjunctiva (lower and/or upper), lacrimal punctum and canaliculi (lower and/or upper), plica, caruncle, posterior eyelid lamella, anterior eyelid lamella and/or eyelid margin (lower and/or upper).

N – Regional Lymph Nodes

NX   Regional lymph nodes cannot be assessed
N0   No regional lymph node metastasis
N1   Regional lymph node metastasis

M – Distant Metastasis

M0   No distant metastasis
M1   Distant metastasis

pTNM Pathological Classification

The pT and pN categories correspond to the T and N categories. For pM see page 8.

Stage

No stage is at present recommended.

Malignant Melanoma of Conjunctiva (ICD-O-3 C69.0)

Rules for Classification

The classification applies only to conjunctival malignant melanoma. There should be histological confirmation of the disease.

The following are the procedures for assessing T, N, and M categories:

T *categories*   Physical examination
N *categories*   Physical examination
M *categories*   Physical examination and imaging

Regional Lymph Nodes

The regional lymph nodes are the preauricular, submandibular, and cervical lymph nodes.

TNM Clinical Classification

T – Primary Tumour

TX   Primary tumour cannot be assessed
T0   No evidence of primary tumour
Tis   Melanoma confined to the conjunctival epithelium (in situ)[a]

T1   Melanoma of the bulbar conjunctiva
    T1a   Tumour involves less than or equal to one quadrant[b]
    T1b   Tumour involves more than one but less than or equal to two quadrants
    T1c   Tumour involves more than two but less than or equal to three quadrants
    T1d   Tumour involves more than three quadrants
T2   Malignant conjunctival melanoma of the non-bulbar conjunctiva involving palpebral, forniceal, and/or caruncular conjunctiva
    T2a   Non-caruncular tumour involves less than or equal to one quadrant
    T2b   Non-caruncular tumour involves more than one quadrant
    T2c   Caruncular tumour involves less than or equal to one quadrant of conjunctiva
    T2d   Caruncular tumour involves more than one quadrant of conjunctiva

T3   Tumour with local invasion into:

    T3a   Globe

    T3b   Eyelid

    T3c   Orbit

    T3d   Paranasal sinus, nasolacrimal duct, and/or lacrimal gland

T4   Tumour invades central nervous system

Notes

[a] Melanoma in situ (includes the term primary acquired melanosis) with atypia replacing greater than 75% of the normal epithelial thickness with cytological features of epithelial cells, including abundant cytoplasm, vesicular nuclei, or prominent nucleoli, and/or presence of intraepithelial nest of atypical cells.

[b] Quadrants are defined by clock hour, starting at the limbus (e.g., 6, 9, 12, 3) extending from the central cornea, to and beyond the eyelid margins. This will bisect the caruncle.

N – Regional Lymph Nodes

NX   Regional lymph nodes cannot be assessed

N0   No regional lymph node metastasis

N1   Regional lymph node metastasis

M – Distant Metastasis

M0   No distant metastasis

M1   Distant metastasis

pTNM Pathological Classification

pT – Primary Tumour

pTX   Primary tumour cannot be assessed

pT0   No evidence of primary tumour

pTis   Melanoma confined to the conjunctival epithelium (in situ)*

pT1   Melanoma of the bulbar conjunctiva

    pT1a   Tumour 2.0 mm or less in thickness with invasion of the substantia propria

    pT1b   Tumour more than 2.0 mm in thickness with invasion of the substantia propria

pT2   Melanoma of the palpebral, forniceal or caruncular conjunctiva

     pT2a   Tumour 2.0 mm or less in thickness with invasion of the substantia propria

     pT2b   Tumour more than 2.0 mm in thickness with invasion of the substantia propria

pT3   Melanoma invades the eye, eyelid, nasolacrimal system or orbit

     pT3a   Invades the globe

     pT3b   Invade the eyelid

     pT3c   Invades the orbit

     pT3d   Invades the paranasal sinus and/or nasolacrimal duct or lacrimal sac

pT4   Melanoma invades central nervous system

Note

* pTis Melanoma in situ (includes the term primary acquired melanosis) with atypia replacing greater than 75 % of the normal epithelial thickness, with cytological features of epithelioid cells, including abundant cytoplasm, vesicular nuclei or prominent nucleoli, and/or presence of intraepithelial nests of atypical cells.

pN – Regional Lymph Nodes

The pN categories correspond to the N categories.

pM – Distant Metastasis

For pM categories see page 8.

G – Histopathological Grading

Histological grade represents the origin of the primary tumour.

GX   Origin cannot be assessed

G0   Primary acquired melanosis without cellular atypia

G1   Conjunctival nevus

G2   Primary acquired melanosis with cellular atypia (epithelial disease only)

G3   Primary acquired melanosis with epithelial cellular atypia and invasive melanoma

G4   De novo malignant melanoma

Stage

No stage is at present recommended.

Malignant Melanoma of Uvea
(ICD-O C69.3,4)

Rules for Classification

There should be histological confirmation of the disease.

The following are the procedures for assessing T, N, and M categories:

T *categories*	Physical examination; additional methods such as fluorescein angiography and isotope examination may enhance the accuracy of appraisal
N *categories*	Physical examination
M *categories*	Examination and imaging

Regional Lymph Nodes

The regional lymph nodes are the preauricular, submandibular, and cervical nodes.

Anatomical Sites

1. Iris (C69.4)
2. Ciliary body (C69.4)
3. Choroid (C69.3)

TNM Clinical Classification

T – Primary Tumour

TX   Primary tumour cannot be assessed
T0   No evidence of primary tumour

*Iris**

T1   Tumour limited to iris
     T1a   not more than 3 clock hours in size
     T1b   more than 3 clock hours in size
     T1c   with secondary glaucoma
T2   Tumour confluent with or extending into the ciliary body, choroid, or both
     T2a   Tumour confluent with or extending into the ciliary body without secondary glaucoma

T2b   Tumour confluent with or extending into the choroid without secondary glaucoma

T2c   Tumour confluent with or extending into the ciliary body and/or choroid with secondary glaucoma

T3   Tumour confluent with or extending into the ciliary body, choroid or both, with scleral extension

T4   Tumour with extrascleral extension

T4a   less than or equal to 5 mm in diameter

T4b   more than 5 mm in diameter

Note

* Iris melanomas originate from, and are predominantly located in, this region of the uvea. If less than half of the tumour volume is located within the iris, the tumour may have originated in the ciliary body and consideration should be given to classifying it accordingly.

Ciliary Body and Choroid

Primary ciliary body and choroidal melanomas are classified according to the four tumour size categories listed in this section.[a, b]

T1   Tumour size category 1

T1a   without ciliary body involvement and extraocular extension

T1b   with ciliary body involvement

T1c   without ciliary body involvement but with extraocular extension less than or equal to 5 mm in diameter

T1d   with ciliary body involvement and extraocular extension less than or equal to 5 mm in diameter

T2   Tumour size category 2

T2a   without ciliary body involvement and extraocular extension

Thickness (mm)

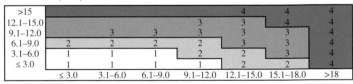

Largest basal diameter (mm)

Figure 1 Classification for ciliary body and choroid uveal melanoma based on thickness and diameter.

T2b with ciliary body involvement

T2c without ciliary body involvement but with extraocular extension less than or equal to 5 mm in diameter

T2d with ciliary body involvement and extraocular extension less than or equal to 5 mm in diameter

T3 Tumour size category 3

T3a without ciliary body involvement and extraocular extension

T3b with ciliary body involvement

T3c without ciliary body involvement but with extraocular extension less than or equal to 5 mm in diameter

T3d with ciliary body involvement and extraocular extension less than or equal to 5 mm in diameter

T4 Tumour size category 4

T4a without ciliary body involvement and extraocular extension

T4b with ciliary body involvement

T4c without ciliary body involvement but with extraocular extension less than or equal to 5 mm in diameter

T4d with ciliary body involvement and extraocular extension less than or equal to 5 mm in diameter

T4e Any tumour size category with extraocular extension more than 5 mm in diameter

Notes

[a] In clinical practice, the largest tumour basal diameter may be estimated in optic disc diameters (dd, average: 1 dd = 1.5 mm). Tumour thickness may be estimated in diopters (average: 2.5 diopters = 1 mm). However, techniques such as ultrasonography and fundus photography are used to provide more accurate measurements. Ciliary body involvement can be evaluated by the slit-lamp, ophthalmoscopy, gonioscopy, and transillumination. However, high-frequency ultrasonography (ultrasound biomicroscopy) is used for more accurate assessment. Extension through the sclera is evaluated visually before and during surgery, and with ultrasonography, computed tomography, or magnetic resonance imaging.

[b] When histopathological measurements are recorded after fixation, tumour diameter and thickness may be underestimated because of tissue shrinkage.

N – Regional Lymph Nodes

NX Regional lymph nodes cannot be assessed

N0 No regional lymph node metastasis

N1 Regional lymph node metastasis

Ophthalmic

M – Distant Metastasis

M0   No distant metastasis
M1   Distant metastasis

 M1a Largest metastases 3 cm or less in greatest dimension
 M1b Largest metastases is larger than 3 cm in greatest dimension but not larger than 8 cm
 M1c Largest metastases is larger than 8 cm in greatest dimension

pTNM Pathological Classification

The pT and pN categories correspond to the T and N categories. For pM see page 8.

Stage

Stage I	T1a	N0	M0
Stage IIA	T1b–d, T2a	N0	M0
Stage IIB	T2b, T3a	N0	M0
Stage IIIA	T2c–d	N0	M0
	T3b–c	N0	M0
	T4a	N0	M0
Stage IIIB	T3d	N0	M0
	T4b–c	N0	M0
Stage IIIC	T4d–e	N0	M0
Stage IV	Any T	N1	M0
	Any T	Any N	M1

Prognostic Factors Grid

Prognostic factors for survival for uveal melanoma

Prognostic factors	Tumour related	Host related	Environment related
Essential	Largest tumour diameter (typically width)	Advanced age	
	Higher UICC T category (associated with worse survival)		
Additional	Extrascleral 'extraocular' extension		
	Location (iris tumours are typically smaller at diagnosis, while ciliary body tumours are less visible and typically larger at diagnosis)		
	Histopathological cell type (spindle cell more favourable than epithelioid)		
	Mitotic activity		
	Microvasculature patterns		
New and promising	PET-CT standardized uptake value (SUV): higher SUV associated with worse prognosis		Immunotherapy
	Monosomy 3, abnormalities of chromosomes 6 and 8*		
	Genetic expression profiling (class 1 more favourable than 1A and 2)		

* Test has been independently confirmed at multiple centres.

Source: UICC Manual of Clinical Oncology, Ninth Edition. Edited by Brian O'Sullivan, James D. Brierley, Anil K. D'Cruz, Martin F. Fey, Raphael Pollock, Jan B. Vermorken and Shao Hui Huang. © 2015 UICC. Published 2015 by John Wiley & Sons, Ltd.

Ophthalmic

Retinoblastoma
(ICD-O-3 C69.2)

Rules for Classification

In bilateral cases, the eyes should be classified separately. The classification does not apply to complete spontaneous regression of the tumour. There should be histological confirmation of the disease in an enucleated eye.

The following are the procedures for assessing T, N, and M categories:

T *categories*   Physical examination and imaging

N *categories*   Physical examination

M *categories*   Physical examination and imaging; examination of bone marrow and cerebrospinal fluid may enhance the accuracy of appraisal

Regional Lymph Nodes

The regional lymph nodes are the preauricular, submandibular, and cervical lymph nodes.

TNM Clinical Classification

T – Primary Tumour

TX   Primary tumour cannot be assessed.

T0   No evidence of primary tumour.

T1   Tumour confined to the retina with subretinal fluid no more than 5 mm from the base of any tumour, without retinal detachment

    T1a   No tumour in either eye is greater than 3 mm in largest dimension or located closer than 1.5 mm to the optic nerve or fovea

    T1b   At least one tumour is greater than 3 mm in largest dimension or located closer than 1.5 mm to the optic nerve or fovea. No retinal detachment or subretinal fluid beyond 5 mm from the base of the tumour

T2   Tumours with vitreous or subretinal seeding or retinal detachment

    T2a   tumour with subretinal fluid more than 5 mm from the base of any tumour

    T2b   Tumour with vitreous and/or subretinal seeding

T3   Severe intraocular disease

    T3a   Phthisis or prephthisis bulbi

T3b Invasion of: choroid, pars plana, ciliary body, lens, zonules, iris or anterior chamber

T3c Raided intraocular pressure with neovascularization and/or buphthalmos

T3d Hyphema and or massive vitreous haemorrhage

T3e Aseptic orbital cellulitis

T4 Extraocular tumour

T4a Invasion of optic nerve or orbital tissues

T4b Extraocular invasion with proptosis and/or orbital mass

N – Regional Lymph Nodes

NX Regional lymph nodes cannot be assessed

N0 No regional lymph node metastasis

N1 Regional lymph node metastasis

M – Distant Metastasis

M0 No distant metastasis

M1 Distant metastasis

M1a Single or multiple metastasis to sites other than CNS or brain

M1b Metastasis to the CNS including brain

TNM Pathological Classification

T – Primary Tumour

pTX Primary tumour cannot be assessed

pT0 No evidence of primary tumour

pT1 Tumour confined to eye with no optic nerve or choroidal invasion

pT2 Tumour with intraocular invasion

pT2a Focal choroidal invasion and pre- or intralaminar invasion of the optic nerve head

pT2b Tumour invasion of stroma of iris and/or trabecular meshwork and/or Schlemm's canal

pT3 Tumour with significant local invasion

pT3a Choroidal invasion larger than 3 mm in diameter or multiple foci of invasion totalling more than 3 mm or any full-thickness involvement

pT3b Retrolaminar invasion of optic nerve without invasion of transected end of optic nerve

pT3c Partial-thickness involvement of sclera within the inner two-thirds

pT3d Full-thickness invasion into outer third of the sclera and/or invasion into or around emissary channels

pT4 Extraocular extension: Tumour invades optic nerve at transected end, in meningeal space around the optic nerve, full-thickness invasion of the sclera with invasion of the episclera, adipose tissue, extraocular muscle, bone, conjunctiva, or eyelid.

N – Regional Lymph Nodes

pNX Regional lymph nodes cannot be assessed

pN0 No regional lymph node involvement

pN1 Regional lymph node involvement

pM – Metastasis

cM0 No distant metastasis

pM1 Distant metastasis

pM1a Single or multiple metastasis to sites other than CNS

pM1b Metastasis to CNS parenchyma or CSF fluid

Stage

Clinical Stage

Stage I	T1,T2,T3	N0	M0
Stage II	T4a	N0	M0
Stage III	T4b	N0	M0
	Any T	N1	M0
Stage IV	Any T	Any N	M1

Pathological Stage

Stage I	T1,T2,T3	N0	M0
Stage II	T4	N0	M0
Stage III	Any T	N1	M0
Stage IV	Any T	Any N	M1

Prognostic Factors Grid

Prognostic factors for survival for retinoblastoma

Prognostic factors	Tumour related	Host related	Environment related
Essential	Massive = > or equal to 3-mm' uveal invasion	Immunosuppression (i.e. AIDS)	Access to care
	Extrascleral tumour extension	Germline mutation	
	Optic nerve invasion	RB1 allele	
	Anterior chamber extension		
	Higher UICC T category		
Additional	Multidrug resistance gene(s)		Cyclosporine therapy
	Heritability		Experienced multidisciplinary team (local control)
New and promising			Screening programmes for less developed countries
			Telepathology for evaluation of enucleated eyes In utero detection of Rb

Source: UICC Manual of Clinical Oncology, Ninth Edition. Edited by Brian O'Sullivan, James D. Brierley, Anil K. D'Cruz, Martin F. Fey, Raphael Pollock, Jan B. Vermorken and Shao Hui Huang. © 2015 UICC. Published 2015 by John Wiley & Sons, Ltd.

Ophthalmic

Sarcoma of Orbit
(ICD-O-3 C69.6)

Rules for Classification

The classification applies to sarcomas of soft tissue and bone. There should be histological confirmation of the disease and division of cases by histological type.

The following are the procedures for assessing T, N, and M categories:

T *categories*   Physical examination and imaging
N *categories*   Physical examination
M *categories*   Physical examination and imaging

Regional Lymph Nodes

The regional lymph nodes are the preauricular, submandibular, and cervical lymph nodes.

TNM Clinical Classification

T – Primary Tumour

TX   Primary tumour cannot be assessed
T0   No evidence of primary tumour

T1   Tumour 20 mm or less in greatest dimension
T2   Tumour more than 20 mm in greatest dimension without invasion of globe or bony wall
T3   Tumour of any size with invasion of orbital tissues and/or bony walls
T4   Tumour invades globe or periorbital structure, such as eyelids, temporal fossa, nasal cavity and paranasal sinuses, and/or central nervous system

N – Regional Lymph Nodes

NX   Regional lymph nodes cannot be assessed
N0   No regional lymph node metastasis
N1   Regional lymph node metastasis

M – Distant Metastasis

M0   No distant metastasis
M1   Distant metastasis

pTNM Pathological Classification

The pT and pN categories correspond to the T and N categories. For pM see page 8.

Stage

No stage is at present recommended.

Carcinoma of Lacrimal Gland (ICD-O-3 C69.5)

Rules for Classification

There should be histological confirmation of the disease and division of cases by histological type.

The following are the procedures for assessing T, N, and M categories:

T *categories*   Physical examination and imaging
N *categories*   Physical examination
M *categories*   Physical examination and imaging

Regional Lymph Nodes

The regional lymph nodes are the preauricular, submandibular, and cervical lymph nodes.

TNM Clinical Classification

T – Primary Tumour

TX   Primary tumour cannot be assessed
T0   No evidence of primary tumour

T1   Tumour 2 cm or less in greatest dimension, with or without extraglandular extension into the orbital soft tissue
  T1a   No periosteal or bone involvement
  T1b   Periosteal involvement with out bone involvement
  T1c   Bone involvement
T2   Tumour more than 2 cm but not more than 4 cm in greatest dimension, limited to the lacrimal gland
  T2a   No periosteal or bone involvement
  T2b   Periosteal involvement without bone involvement
  T2c   Bone involvement
T3   Tumour more than 4 cm or with extraglandular extension into orbital soft tissue, including optic nerve, or globe
  T3a   No periosteal or bone involvement
  T3b   Periosteal involvement without bone involvement
  T3c   Bone involvement

T4   Tumour invades adjacent structures (sinuses, temporal fossa, ptery-
     goid fossa, superior orbital fissure, cavernous sinus, and/or brain)

     T4a   No more than 2 cm in greatest dimension
     T4b   More than 2 cm but no more than 4 cm in greatest dimension
     T4c   More than 4 cm in greatest dimension

N – Regional Lymph Nodes

NX   Regional lymph nodes cannot be assessed
N0   No regional lymph node metastasis
N1   Regional lymph node metastasis

M – Distant Metastasis

M0   No distant metastasis
M1   Distant metastasis

pTNM Pathological Classification

The pT and pN categories correspond to the T and N categories. For pM
see page 8.

Stage

No stage is at present recommended.

Ophthalmic

Hodgkin Lymphoma

Introductory Notes

The current staging classification for Hodgkin Lymphoma is a modification of the Ann Arbor classification first adopted in 1971. Over the past 45 years the practice has changed, making the previously used staging laparotomy and the resulting pathological staging classification obsolete. The recent consensus conference that took place in 2012 in Lugano suggested even more simplified system putting together stage I and II as Limited Stage and stage III and IV as Advanced Stage lymphoma. The Lugano Classification, a modification of the Ann Arbor classification, has been published and accepted by the UICC.[1]

Clinical Staging (cS)

It is determined by history, clinical examination, imaging, blood analysis, and the initial biopsy report. Bone marrow biopsy must be taken from a clinically or radiologically non-involved area of bone.

Liver Involvement
Clinical evidence of liver involvement must include either enlargement of the liver and at least an abnormal serum alkaline phosphatase level and two different liver function test abnormalities, or an abnormal liver demonstrated by imaging and one abnormal liver function test.

Spleen Involvement
Clinical evidence of spleen involvement is accepted if there is palpable enlargement of the spleen confirmed by imaging.

Lymphatic and Extralymphatic Disease
The lymphatic structures are as follows:
- Lymph nodes
- Waldeyer ring

Hodgkin

TNM Classification of Malignant Tumours, Eighth Edition. Edited by James D. Brierley, Mary K. Gospodarowicz and Christian Wittekind.
© 2017 UICC. Published 2017 by John Wiley & Sons, Ltd.

- Spleen
- Appendix
- Thymus
- Peyer patches

The lymph nodes are grouped into regions and one or more (2, 3, etc.) may be involved. The spleen is designated S and extralymphatic organs or sites E.

Lung Involvement

Lung involvement limited to one lobe, or perihilar extension associated with ipsilateral lymphadenopathy, or unilateral pleural effusion with or without lung involvement but with hilar lymphadenopathy is considered as **localized** extralymphatic disease.

Liver Involvement

Liver involvement is always considered as **diffuse** extralymphatic disease.

Clinical Stages (cS)

Limited Stage

Stage I

Involvement of a single lymph node region (I), or localized involvement of a single extralymphatic organ or site (IE).

Stage II

Involvement of two or more lymph node regions on the same side of the diaphragm (II), or localized involvement of a single extralymphatic organ or site and its regional lymph node(s) with or without involvement of other contiguous lymph node regions on the same side of the diaphragm (IIE).

Bulky Stage II

Stage II disease with a single nodal mass greater than 10 cm in maximum dimension or greater than a third of the thoracic diameter as assessed on CT.

Advanced Stage

Stage III

Involvement of lymph node regions on both sides of the diaphragm (III), which may also be accompanied by involvement of the spleen (IIIS).

Stage IV
Disseminated (multifocal) involvement of one or more extralymphatic organs, with or without associated lymph node involvement; or non-contiguous extralymphatic organ involvement with involvement of lymph node regions on the same or both sides of the diaphragm.

A and B Classification (Symptoms)
Each stage should be divided into A and B according to the absence or presence of defined general symptoms. These are:
1. Unexplained weight loss of more than 10% of the usual body weight in the 6 months prior to first attendance
2. Unexplained fever with temperature above 38 °C
3. Night sweats

Note
Pruritus alone does not qualify for B classification nor does a short, febrile illness associated with a known infection.

Reference

1 Cheson BD, Fisher RI, Barrington SF, et al. Recommendations for initial evaluation, staging, and response assessment of Hodgkin and non-Hodgkin lymphoma: the Lugano classification. *J Clin Oncol* 2014; 32: 3059–3068.

Hodgkin

Non-Hodgkin Lymphomas

The Lugano classification, a modification of the Ann Arbor classification, is recommended as for Hodgkin lymphoma with the exception of the elimination of the A or B classification of symptoms (see page 237).

In Stage II disease, bulk is defined as larger than 6 cm in greatest dimension in follicular lymphoma, and 10 cm in largest dimension has been recommended for diffuse large cell lymphoma.

TNM Classification of Malignant Tumours, Eighth Edition. Edited by James D. Brierley, Mary K. Gospodarowicz and Christian Wittekind.
© 2017 UICC. Published 2017 by John Wiley & Sons, Ltd.

Non-Hodgkin Lymphomas

Essential TNM

Introductory Notes (see also page 13)

When the T, N, and M categories have not been recorded in the clinical records or if the data to determine the categories is not available, the cancer registrar can code the extent of disease according to the Essential TNM scheme. Using the schema for breast, colorectal, prostate, or cervical cancer (Figures 2, 3, 4, and 5), the extent of disease may be recorded as Stage I, II, III, or IV or if insufficient data as distant, regional, or localized.

Rules for Classification

Essential TNM is composed of three key elements that together summarize the extent of cancer in the patient:

M Presence or absence of distant metastasis

N Presence or absence of regional lymph node metastasis/involvement

T Extent of invasion and/or size of the tumour

Coding the Elements of Essential TNM

Metastasis (M)

M+ Presence of distant metastasis including non-regional nodes

M− No mention of distant metastases, clinically or pathologically

Regional Node Metastasis/Involvement (N)

R+ Presence of regional node metastasis/involvement

R− No mention of regional node metastases, clinically or pathologically

TNM Classification of Malignant Tumours, Eighth Edition. Edited by James D. Brierley, Mary K. Gospodarowicz and Christian Wittekind.
© 2017 UICC. Published 2017 by John Wiley & Sons, Ltd.

Extent of Invasion and/or Size of Tumour (T)

Depending on the information available, the T category can be recorded or if not available the extent of the local tumour as advanced or localized.

A   Extent of invasion and/or tumour size is **Advanced**

    A2   Extent of invasion and/or tumour size is very advanced

    A1   Extent of invasion and/or tumour size is advanced

L   Extent of invasion and/or tumour size is **Limited**

    L2   Extent of invasion and/or tumour size is limited

    L1   Extent of invasion and/or tumour size is very limited

X   Extent of invasion and/or tumour size cannot be assessed

Colon and Rectum Essential TNM

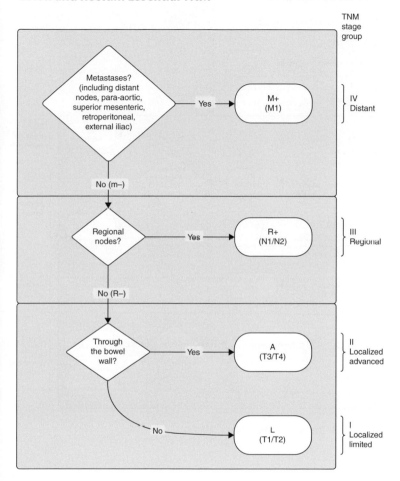

Figure 2 Colon and rectum essential TNM.

Breast Essential TNM

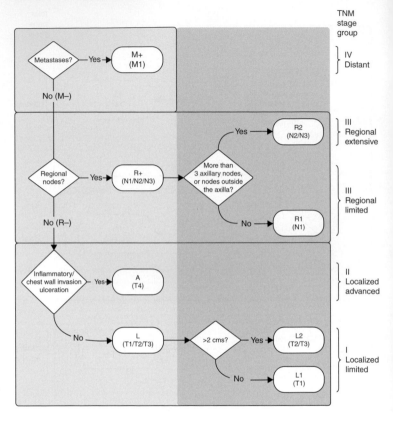

Figure 3 Breast essential TNM.

Cervix Essential TNM

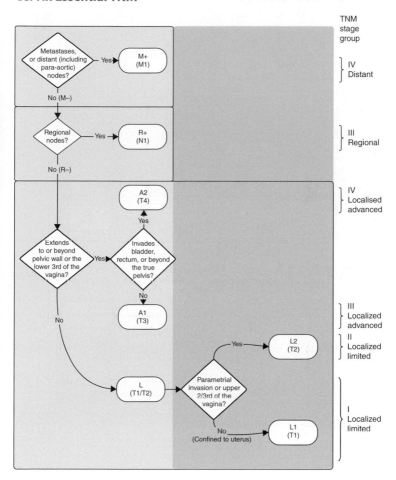

Figure 4 Cervix essential TNM.

Prostate Essential TNM

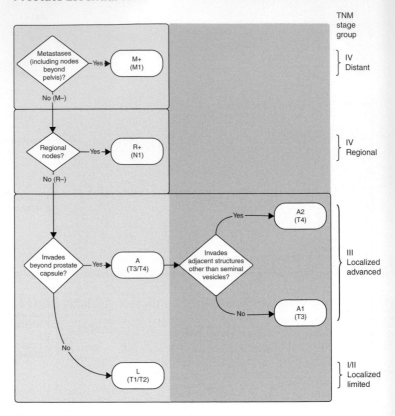

Figure 5 Prostate essential TNM.

Paediatric Tumours

Introductory Notes (see also page 13)

The classifications in this section are not intended to replace the classifications used by the clinician when treating an individual patient but to facilitate the collection of stage by population-based cancer registries. The consensus meeting held in 2014 recommended a tiered staging system with more-detailed systems for well-resourced cancer registries and less-detailed systems for registries with limited recourses and access; as with Essential TNM, lower-tiered systems are based on collapsing higher-tiered systems.[1] The recommendations for tier 1 and 2 follow. Well-resourced registries may choose to collect additional accepted prognostic factors such as those used in the clinical setting but these are not included in this section. For some cancers, recommendations are the same as described earlier for adult patients and the appropriate page number is given; others are referenced where appropriate. Rules for the derivation of paediatric cancer stage in population-based cancer registries are being developed and will be available from the UICC website when available.[2]

Rules for Classification

The classification applies only to paediatric malignant tumours.

Gastrointestinal Tumours

Hepatoblastoma

Tier 1 and 2

Metastatic	Distant metastases present
Localized	Tumour confined to the liver including regional lymph nodes

Well-resourced cancer registries may wish to use the Pretext Classification.[3]

TNM Classification of Malignant Tumours, Eighth Edition. Edited by James D. Brierley, Mary K. Gospodarowicz and Christian Wittekind.

Paediatric

Bone and Soft Tissue Tumours

Osteosarcoma

Tier 1 and 2

Metastatic   Distant metastases present

Localized   Tumour confined to area of origin including regional lymph nodes

Ewing Sarcoma

Tier 1 and 2

Metastatic   Distant metastases present

Localized   Tumour confined to area of origin including regional lymph nodes

Rhabdomyosarcoma

Tier 1

Metastatic   Distant metastases present

Localized   Tumour confined to the area of origin including regional lymph nodes

Tier 2

A modified TNM Clinical Classification with the addition of favourable or non-favourable tumour site.

T – Primary Tumour*

TX   Primary tumour cannot be assessed
T0   No evidence of primary tumour

T1   Confined to a single anatomic site
T1a   Tumour 5 cm or less in greatest dimension
T1b   Tumour more than 5 cm in greatest dimension
T2   Extension beyond anatomic site
T2a   Tumour 5 cm or less in greatest dimension
T2b   Tumour more than 5 cm in greatest dimension

N – Regional Lymph Nodes

NX   Regional lymph nodes cannot be assessed
N0   No regional lymph node metastasis
N1   Regional lymph node metastasis

M – Distant Metastasis

M0   No distant metastasis
M1   Distant metastasis

Note
*For the eighth edition in adults this has been revised (see page 124).

Prognostic Grouping

The prognostic grouping for rhabdomyosarcoma includes favourable anatomic sites and unfavourable anatomic sites.

Favourable anatomic sites: Orbit, head and neck(excluding parameningeal tumours) and genitourinary sites (excluding bladder and prostate tumours)

Unfavourable anatomic sites: Bladder, prostate, extremity, cranial, parameningeal, trunk, retroperitoneum and all other sites not noted as favourable

Stage I	Any T	Any N	M0	Favourable Site
Stage II	T1a, T2a	N0	M0	Unfavourable Site
Stage III	T1a, T2a	N1	M0	Unfavourable Site
	T1b, T2b	Any N	M0	Unfavourable Site
Stage IV	Any T	Any N	M1	Any Site

Soft Tissue Sarcoma other than Rhabdomyosarcoma

Tier 1

> Metastatic   Distant metastases present
> Localized   Tumour confined to the area of origin including regional lymph nodes

Tier 2

> The TNM Classification is recommended

See Classification for soft tissue sarcoma of the trunk and extremity on page 124 for definitions of T category and N category.

Gynaecological Tumours

Ovary*

Tier 1

> Metastatic   Distant metastases excluding peritoneal metastases

Regional   Tumour extension to pelvis, peritoneum outside the pelvis, and/or retroperitoneal lymph nodes

Localized   Tumour confined to the ovaries (one or both)

Tier 2

Stage I   Tumour confined to the ovaries (one or both)

Stage II   Tumour extension to pelvis without extension to perito-neum outside the pelvis nor to retroperitoneal lymph nodes

Stage III   Tumour extension to peritoneum outside the pelvis and/or retroperitoneal lymph nodes

Stage IV   Distant metastases present (excludes peritoneal metastases)

Note

* The UICC Stage Group corresponds to the FIGO stage.

Urological Tumours

Testes

Tier 1

Metastatic   Distant metastases present

Regional   Tumour extension to regional lymph nodes

Localized   Tumour confined to the testes

Tier 2

See Classification for testes on page 195 for definitions of T category and N category.*

Stage I	Any T	N0	M0
Stage II	Any T	N1, N2, N3	M0
Stage III	Any T	Any N	M1

Note

* For Tier 2 this is irrespective of serum tumour markers.

Well-resourced cancer registries may wish to use the Classification on page 195 as used for adults that includes serum tumour markers.

Wilms Tumour

Tier 1

Metastatic   Distant metastases present
Localized   Tumour confined to the area of origin

Tier 2

Two Tier 2 staging classifications exist for Wilms Tumour. The classification of the Children's Oncology Group/National Wilms Tumour Study Group (NWTSG) is utilized after surgical resection, prior to chemotherapy. The classification of the International Society of Paediatric Oncology (SIOP) is utilized if chemotherapy has been given preoperatively, prior to surgical resection.[4]

Ophthalmic Tumours

Retinoblastoma

Tier 1

Metastatic   Distant metastases present
Regional   Orbital extension or regional lymph nodes
Localized   Intraocular

Tier 2

This classification is determined after enucleation and is therefore a pathological classification.

Prognostic Group

Stage 0   The tumour is confined to the globe. Enucleation has not been performed
pStage I   Enucleation with negative margins (R0)
pStage II   Enucleation with microscopic residual disease (R1)
pStage III   Involvement of the orbit and/or metastases to regional lymph nodes
cStage IV   Metastatic disease

Note

Well-resourced cancer registries may wish to use the Classification page 226 as used for adults.

Malignant Lymphoma

Hodgkin Lymphoma

See Classification on page 235.

Non-Hodgkin Lymphoma

Tier 1

Advanced	Involvement of bone marrow and/or CNS
Limited	No involvement of bone marrow or CNS

Tier 2

The St Jude/Murphy system is recommended[5]

Stage I	Involvement of a single tumour mass or nodal area, excluding the mediastinum and abdomen
Stage II	Involvement of a single tumour mass with regional node(s) or two or more tumours and/or nodal regions on the same side of the diaphragm, or a completely resected primary gastrointestinal tract tumour with or without regional nodal involvement
Stage III	Tumour masses and/or regional nodes on opposite sides of the diaphragm or primary intrathoracic tumour (mediastinal, pleural or thymic) or extensive primary intra-abdominal disease or paraspinal tumour or epidural tumour
Stage IV	Involvement of bone marrow and/or central nervous system

Central Nervous System

Medulloblastoma and Ependymoma

Tier 1

Metastatic	Disease beyond local site (e.g., other lesions in brain or spine, tumour cells in CSF or distant metastases)
Localized	Localized disease

Tier 2

The classification is based on the extent of metastatic disease.[6]

Neuroblastoma

Tier 1

MS	Metastatic disease confined to skin, liver and/or bone marrow in a patient less than 18 months of age
Metastatic	Distant metastatic disease except stage MS
Locoregional	More extensive without metastatic disease
Localized	Localized not involving vital structures and confined to one body site

Tier 2

The stage classification of the International Neuroblastoma Risk Group Staging System (INRGSS) is recommended.[7]

References

1 Gupta S, Aitken J, Bartels U, et al. Paediatric cancer stage in population-based cancer registries: the Toronto consensus principles and guidelines. *Lancet Oncol* 2016; 17: 163–172.
2 Aitken JF, Youlden DR, Ward LJ, et al. *Rules for Derivation of Paediatric Cancer Stage in Population-Based Cancer Registries, according to the Toronto Consensus Principles and Guidelines.* Brisbane, Australia: Viertel Cancer Research Centre, Cancer Council Queensland, in press.
3 Roebuck DJ, Aronson D, Clapuyt P, et al. 2005 PRETEXT: a revised staging system for primary malignant liver tumours of childhood developed by the SIOPEL group. *Pediatric Radiol* 2007; 37. 123–132.
4 Metzger ML, Dome JS. Current therapy for Wilms' tumor. *Oncologist* 2005; 10: 815–826.
5 Murphy SB. Classification, staging and end results of treatment of childhood non-Hodgkin's lymphomas: dissimilarities from lymphomas in adults. *Semin Oncol* 1980; 7: 332–339.
6 Harisiadis L, Chang CH. Medulloblastoma in children: a correlation between staging and results of treatment. *Int J Radiation Oncol Biol Phys* 1977; 2: 833–841.
7 Monclair T, Brodeur GM, Ambros PF, et al. and the INRG Task Force. The International Neuroblastoma Risk Group (INRG) staging system: an INRG Task Force report. *J Clin Oncol* 2009; 27: 298–303.

Paediatric